ENTRANCE EXAMINATION IN HAEMATOLOGY

(Includes Important Text, Original solved MCQ's and their Explanations)

Editor

Dr. M.S. Bhatia

M.D., F.I.P., Dip. W.P.A., M.N.A.M.S.

Prof. & Head, Department of Psychiatry,
University College of Medical Sciences &
Guru Teg Bahadur Hospital,
Dilshad Garden, Delhi - 110 095 (India)

Contributing Editor

Dr. (Mrs.) Nirmaljit Kaur M.D.

Senior Specialist, Department of Microbiology,
Dr. R.M.L. Hospital,
New Delhi - 110 001 (India)

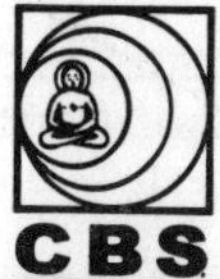

CBS Publishers & Distributors Pvt. Ltd.

New Delhi • Bengaluru • Chennai • Kochi • Kolkata • Mumbai
Hyderabad • Nagpur • Patna • Pune • Vijayawada

Dedicated to
Respected Teachers
&
Beloved Students

ISBN: 978-81-239-1792-4
First Edition: 2009
Reprint: 2017

Published by **Satish Kumar Jain** and produced by **Varun Jain** for
CBS Publishers & Distributors Pvt. Ltd.,
4819/XI Prahlad Street, 24 Ansari Road, Daryaganj, New Delhi - 110002
delhi@cbspd.com, cbspubs@airtelmail.in • www.cbspd.com
Ph.: 23289259, 23266861, 23266867 • Fax: 011-23243014

Corporate Office: 204 FIE, Industrial Area, Patparganj, Delhi - 110 092
Ph: 49344934 • Fax: 011-49344935
E-mail: publishing@cbspd.com • publicity@cbspd.com

Branches:

- ***Bengaluru:*** 2975, 17th Cross, K.R. Road, Bansankari 2nd Stage, Bengaluru - 70 • Ph: +91-80-26771678/79 • Fax: +91-80-26771680 E-mail: cbsbng@gmail.com, bangalore@cbspd.com
- ***Chennai:*** No. 7, Subbaraya Street, Shenoy Nagar, Chennai - 600030 Ph: +91-44-26681266, 26680620 • Fax: +91-44-42032115 E-mail: chennai@cbspd.com
- ***Kochi:*** Ashana House, 39/1904, A.M. Thomas Road, Valanjambalam, Ernakulum, Kochi • Ph: +91-484-4059061-65 Fax: +91-484-4059065 • E-mail: cochin@cbspd.com
- ***Kolkata:*** 6-B, Ground Floor, Rameshwar Shaw Road, Kolkata - 700014 Ph: +91-33-22891126/7/8 • E-mail: kolkata@cbspd.com
- ***Mumbai:*** 83-C, Dr. E. Moses Road, Worli, Mumbai - 400018 Ph: +91-9833017933, 022-24902340/41 • E-mail: mumbai@cbspd.com

Representatives:

- Hyderabad: 0-9885175004
- Nagpur: 0-9021734563
- Patna: 0-9334159340
- Pune: 0-9623451994
- Vijayawada: 0-9000660880

Printed at:
J.S. Offset Printers, Delhi (India)

PREFACE

Medical science is a rapidly advancing field. Its new allied branches are coming up. In a competitive examination, more and more emphasis is being laid on these allied disciplines. But most of the standard textbooks of Haematology have failed to devote adequate space to these new disciplines.

This book has been written with the aim to outline the major areas of Haematology i.e. Factual data, Biochemical, Physiological, Pharmacological, Pathological and Clinical Aspects and *Recent advances*. This book is not merely an addition to the existing list of books on MCQ's but a sincere ambition and an honest attempt to make it a useful and practical companion to both medical graduates and postgraduates. The present book consists of original solved MCQ's from the *Question Banks* of various important examinations (AIIMS, Delhi, PGI etc.), Important text, original solved MCQ's and their explanations have been added. We hope that this will help the candidates in performing better in the examination.

All suggestions for the modification of this book are welcome and will be duly acknowledged.

—Editors

CONTENTS

Preface v

Dedication

BIOCHEMICAL ASPECTS

IMPORTANT TEXT 1—2

MCQ'S 3—13

EXPLANATIONS 14—20

PHYSIOLOGICAL ASPECTS

IMPORTANT TEXT 21—22

MCQ'S 23—51

EXPLANATIONS 52—69

PHARMACOLOGICAL ASPECTS

IMPORTANT TEXT 70—72

MCQ'S 73—78

EXPLANATIONS 79—80

PATHOLOGICAL ASPECTS

IMPORTANT TEXT 81—84

MCQ'S 85—122

EXPLANATIONS 123—140

CLINICAL ASPECTS

IMPORTANT TEXT 141—142

MCQ'S 143—205

EXPLANATIONS 206—235

REVIEW PAPERS 236—241

BIOCHEMICAL ASPECTS

IMPORTANT TEXT FOR BIOCHEMICAL ASPECTS

CLOTTING FACTORS

Factors	*Name*	*Synthesis*	*Other features*
I	Fibrinogen	Liver	Soluble glycoprotein, Mol. Wt - 340,000 made up of 6 polypeptide chains
II	Prothrombin	Liver	Single chain glycoprotein, Mol. Wt - 72,000
IV	Calcium ions	Absorbed from diet	Required for several stages
V	Labile factor, Proacceleren, Accelerator globin		Does not have any enzyme properties
VII	Proconvertin, Serum Prothrombin Conversion Accelerator (SPCA)		Activated by thrombin
VIII	Antihemophilic globulin (von willebrand factor)		Enhances rate of activation of factor IV
IX	Christmas factor		Converts factor X to Xa
X	Stuart factor		Junction point for extrinsic and intrinsic pathway is a serine protease
XI	Plasma thromboplastin Antecedent (PTA)		Activates factor IX to IXa
XII	Hageman factor		Activated to XIIa by glass or kallikrein

Contd......

CLOTTING FACTORS (Contd....)

Factors	*Name*	*Synthesis*	*Other features*
XIII	Fibrin stabilizing factor (Laki-Lorand factor)		Zymogen form of a transglutaminase Helps consolidation of clot
XIV	Protein C		Zymogen of a protease inactivates factor V and VII
	Pre-kallikrein		On conversion to kallikrein, activates factor XI and XII
	High Mol. Wt. kininogen		Accessory protein factor for activation of factors XI & XII

DIFFERENCES IN REDUCED AND OXIDISED Hb

	T(Taut) form (reduced Hb)	*R(relaxed) form (Oxy Hb)*
1.	$\alpha_1 \beta_2$ and $\alpha_1 \beta_2$ units have their long axis close	There is rotation of 15° between the two
2.	Salt bridges are numerous	Salt bridges less in number
3.	Fe^{++} is 0.07 nm out of the plane of porphyrin ring	Fe^{++} in the plane
4.	Valine residue projects into home pocket of beta chains	Valine residue does not project. Home pocket free to take up O_2
5.	Affinity for O_2 is low	High by several hundred fold
6.	Beta chain histidine residues are protonated (H^+ added)	Histidine of beta chains release proteins ($2H^+$)
7.	DPG can enter and is retained by salt bridges in a central	DPG cannot bind

MCQ'S FOR BIOCHEMICAL ASPECTS

1. **What is the most acute effect of smoking cessation ?** **AIIMS 2005**
   - A. Shift of oxyhemoglobin curve to the right
   - B. Increased ciliary function
   - C. Decreased mucous production
   - D. Decreased incidence of post-operative pneumonia
2. **Which of the following can be a homologous substitution for valine in hemoglobin ?** **AI 2004**
   - A. Isoleucine
   - B. Glutamic acid
   - C. Phenylalanine
   - D. Lysine
3. **Hair is rich in amino acid :** **AIIMS 1983, 87, 94**
   - A. Cystine
   - B. Lysine
   - C. Glycine
   - D. Leucine
4. **Iron in haemoglobin exists as :** **AIIMS 1985, 89**
   - A. Unionised iron atoms
   - B. Ferric irons only
   - C. Ferrous ions only
   - D. None of the above
5. **In sickle cell anaemia, there is fault in which component of haemoglobin is :** **PGI 1983, 96**
   - A. Alpha chain of globin
   - B. Beta chain of globin
   - C. Iron
   - D. Porphyrin
6. **Which of the following is seen in obstructive jaundice?** **AIIMS 1982, 84, 91**
   - A. Excess of urobilinogen in urine
   - B. Excess of unconjugated serum bilirubin
   - C. Excess of bile salts in the urine
   - D. All of these
7. **The blood concentration of H_2CO_3 (meq/L) is :** **Delhi 1984, UPSC 1991**
   - A. 5
   - B. 15
   - C. 28
   - D. 50

Ans. **1. A** **2. B** **3. A** **4. C** **5. B** **6. C** **7. C**

8. During RBC destruction : AIIMS 1983; Delhi 1985, 97

A. Amino acids are excreted and iron preserved
B. Vice versa of above
C. Both are excreted
D. Both are preserved

9. Bohr's effect is : AIIMS 1982, 84, 85, 87; PGI 1988, 92

A. Effect of Zn^{++} on carbonic anhydrase activity
B. Effect of pCO_2 on oxyhemoglobin
C. $HCO3^-$leaving the RBC in exchange of Cl^-
D. H^+ leaving RBC for each CO_2 that enters

10. Chloride shift is : AIIMS 1983, 86; AMC 1986; UPSC 1982, 88, 96

A. HCO_3^- leaving the RBC in exchange for Cl^-
B. CT leaving the RBC in exchange of HCO_3
C. H_2CO_3 leaving the RBC
D. H^+ leaving RBC for each CO_2 that enters

11. Mature RBC contains all except : AIIMS 1984, 91

A. Enzymes of HMP shunt B. Enzymes of TCA cycle
C. Glycolytic enzymes D. Pyridine nucleotides

12. The anticoagulant normally present in animal cell is : PGI 1985, 98

A. Vitamin-K B. Heparin
C. Hyaluronidase D. None of the above

13. Which of the following is not a part of hemoglobin molecule : AIIMS 1983, 92

A. ·Pyrrole rings B. Vinyl rings
C. Histidine D. Ferric ions

14. Protein and lipopolysaccharides are carried in blood is : AMC 1984; Delhi 1986, 89, 97

A. LDL B. HDL
C. VLDL D. Chylomicron

15. Heparin, an anticoagulant substance produced by the mast cells of the liver consists of : AP 1993

A. Acetylated D-Glucosamine and D-Glucuronic acid
B. Sulphated Glucasamine and galactosamine
C. Acetylated galactosamine and glucuronic acid
D. Sulphated D-Glucosamine and D-Glucuronic acid

Ans. 8. A 9. B 10. A 11. B 12. B 13. D 14. B 15. D

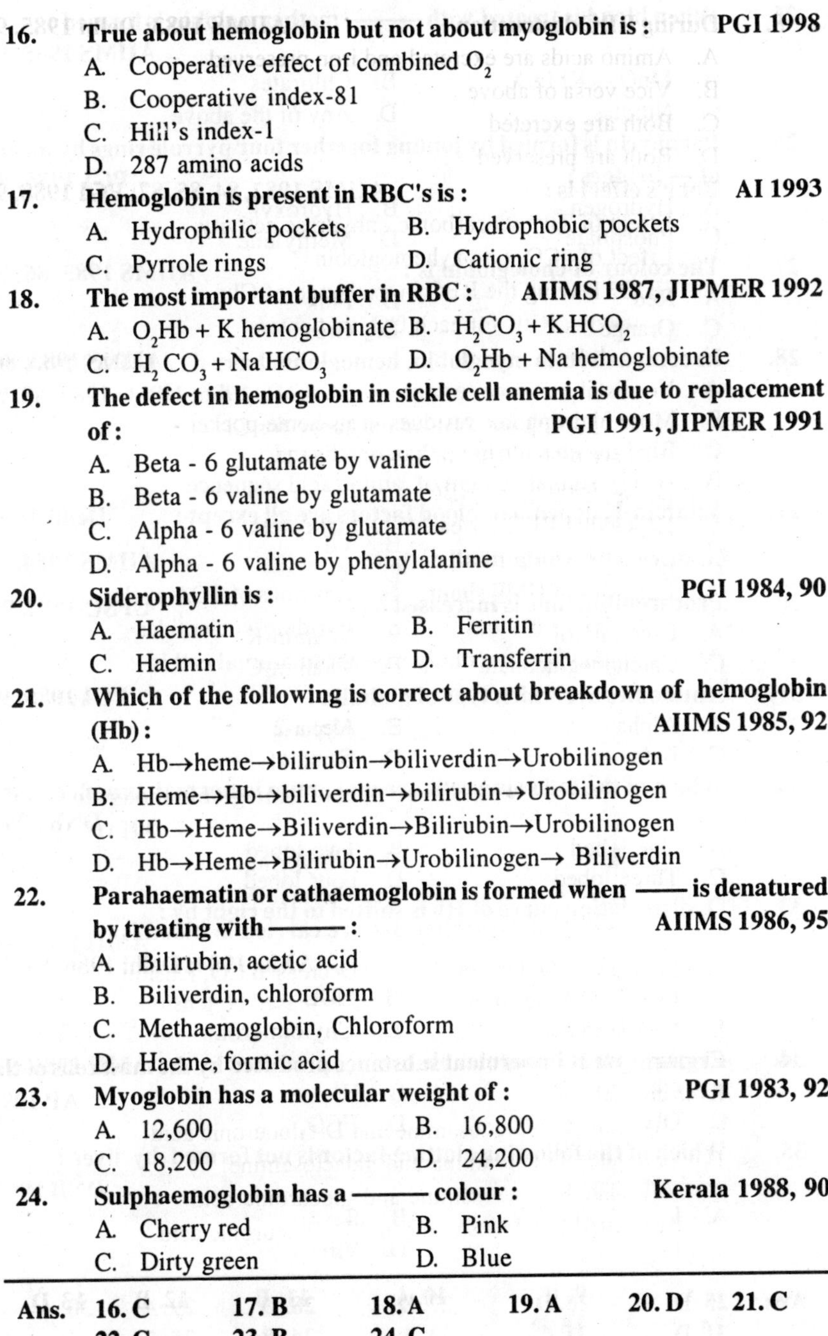

16. True about hemoglobin but not about myoglobin is : **PGI 1998**

A. Cooperative effect of combined O_2

B. Cooperative index-81

C. Hill's index-1

D. 287 amino acids

17. Hemoglobin is present in RBC's is : **AI 1993**

A. Hydrophilic pockets B. Hydrophobic pockets

C. Pyrrole rings D. Cationic ring

18. The most important buffer in RBC : **AIIMS 1987, JIPMER 1992**

A. O_2Hb + K hemoglobinate B. $H_2CO_3 + KHCO_2$

C. $H_2CO_3 + NaHCO_3$ D. O_2Hb + Na hemoglobinate

19. The defect in hemoglobin in sickle cell anemia is due to replacement of : **PGI 1991, JIPMER 1991**

A. Beta - 6 glutamate by valine

B. Beta - 6 valine by glutamate

C. Alpha - 6 valine by glutamate

D. Alpha - 6 valine by phenylalanine

20. Siderophyllin is : **PGI 1984, 90**

A. Haematin B. Ferritin

C. Haemin D. Transferrin

21. Which of the following is correct about breakdown of hemoglobin (Hb) : **AIIMS 1985, 92**

A. Hb→heme→bilirubin→biliverdin→Urobilinogen

B. Heme→Hb→biliverdin→bilirubin→Urobilinogen

C. Hb→Heme→Biliverdin→Bilirubin→Urobilinogen

D. Hb→Heme→Bilirubin→Urobilinogen→ Biliverdin

22. Parahaematin or cathaemoglobin is formed when —— is denatured by treating with ——— : **AIIMS 1986, 95**

A. Bilirubin, acetic acid

B. Biliverdin, chloroform

C. Methaemoglobin, Chloroform

D. Haeme, formic acid

23. Myoglobin has a molecular weight of : **PGI 1983, 92**

A. 12,600 B. 16,800

C. 18,200 D. 24,200

24. Sulphaemoglobin has a ——— colour : **Kerala 1988, 90**

A. Cherry red B. Pink

C. Dirty green D. Blue

Ans. **16. C** **17. B** **18. A** **19. A** **20. D** **21. C**
22. C **23. B** **24. C**

25. **When blood is treated with ——— methemoglobin is formed :** **AIIMS 1985, 93**
A. MnO_4—$KMnO_4$ B. Chlorates
C. Nitrates D. Any of the above

26. **Porphyrin is formed by joining together four pyrrole rings by means of — bridges :** **PGI 1985, 95**
A. Hydrogen B. Hydroxyl
C. Phosphate D. Methylene

27. **The colour of choleglobin is :** **AIIMS 1983, 86, 99**
A. Red B. Pink
C. Orange D. Green

28. **In comparison to myoglobin, hemoglobin has :** **AIIMS 1984, 92**
A. No distal histidine residue
B. More hydrophobic residues in its heme pocket
C. Binding sites for more than one ligand
D. A very similar subunit of amino acid sequence

29. **Vitamin-K dependent blood factors are all except :** **Delhi 1994**
A. V B. VII
C. IX D. X

30. **Prothrombin time is increased by :** **UPSC 1984, 93**
A. Dicoumarol B. Vitamin-K
C. Calcium gluconate D. Vitamin-C

31. **Antibodies are which type of globulin :** **WB 1999**
A. Alpha B. Alpha-2
C. Beta D. Gamma

32. **Which of the following cells are maximum in normal Arneth count :** **DNB 1992**
A. One lobed B. Two lobed
C. Three lobed D. Four lobed

33. **O_2 dissociation curve of Hb is shifted to the right by :** **AMU 1987, 98**
A. Increased CO_2 tension B. Decreased CO_2 tension
C. Increased N_2 tension D. Decreased N_2 tension
E. Increased pH

34. **Erythrocyte is impermeable to :** **AMU 1986, 91**
A. Cl^- B. H^+
C. OH^- D. HCO_3^-

35. **Which of the following clotting factor is not formed by liver :** **DNB 1991**
A. I B. II
C. IV D. VIII

Ans. 25. D 26. D 27. D 28. D 29. A 30. A
31. D 32. C 33. A 34. B 35. C

36. Oxy hemoglobin in comparison to reduced Hb has the following except : PGI 1986, 97

A. Salt bridges are numerous
B. Valine residue does not project
C. DPG can not bind
D. There is rotation of 15° between two subunits

37. Laki-Lorand factor is another name for clotting factor : AIIMS 1986, 93

A. XI B. XII
C. XIII D. XIV

38. Fibrinogen is made up of——— polypeptide chains : UPSC 1982, 98

A. 2 B. 4
C. 6 D. 8

39. Cyclic tetrapyrrole is a synonym of : CMC 1987, 91

A. Heme B. Porphyrin
C. Hemosiderin D. Bilirubin

40. Normal volume index of blood is : DNB 1992

A. 0.4-0.8 B. 0.8-1.1
C. 1.1-1.5 D. 1.5-2.0

41. Bilirubin : Manipal 1995

A. Is a steroid pigment
B. Is carried dissolved (in an unbound form) in the plasma
C. Contains Iron
D. None of the above

42. In haemoglobin "S" the substitution of polar amino acid (Glutamic acid) with the non-polar amino acid (Valine) generates a "Sticky Patch" on the surface of the : Karnataka 1998

A. Alpha chain B. Beta chain
C. Gamma chain D. Delta chain

43. Which of the following proteases is synthesized by the kidney and promotes the breakdown or lysis of blood clots ? AIIMS 1980, 88, 93

A. Urokinase B. Streptokinase
C. Factor-VII D. Plasmin

44. The normal pH of blood is : AIIMS 1983; 84, 87; Delhi 1983, 87; PGI 1983, 99

A. 6.8 B. 7.1
C. 7.4 D. 7.9

Ans. **36. A** **37. C** **38. C** **39. B** **40. B** **41. D**
42. B **43. A** **44. C**

45. Degradation of haemoglobin takes place mainly in : **AIIMS 1984, 90, 99**

A. Kidney tubules
B. Liver parenchyma
C. RBC's
D. Reticuloendothelial system

46. Haemoglobin is responsible ——— % CO_2 transport in blood : **AIIMS 1984; AP 1987, 97**

A. 40
B. 70
C. 90
D. 99

47. Ferritin an inactive form of iron is stored in : **AMC 1982; Delhi 1983, 87, 90**

A. Gut
B. Spleen
C. Liver
D. All of the above

48. Iron absorption is increased by : **UPSC 1984; Delhi 1987, 92**

A. Antacids
B. Calcium
C. Bile salts
D. Ascorbic acid

49. Colour index of blood is : **AIIMS 1986, 93**

A. 0.1-05
B. 0.6-0.9
C. 0.9-1.0
D. 1.0-1.2

50. Cabot's rings in RBC's are typically seen in : **Kerala 1987, 96**

A. Acquired Hemolytic anemia
B. After splenectomy
C. Haemochromatosis
D. Thalassemia

51. Haeme in hemoglobin is : **AIIMS 1983, 99**

A. Between Helix C and D
B. Surrounded by non-polar environment
C. Bonded to E-7 histidine
D. Protoporphyrin-IX

52. Uroporphyrin-III : **AIIMS 1986, 91, 98**

A. Is an intermediate in the biosynthesis of heme
B. Does not contain a tetrapyrrole ring
C. Differs from coproporphyrin-III in the substituents around the ring
D. Is formed from uroporphyrinogen-III by an oxidase

53. One of the following conditions cause excessive accumulation of Ketone bodies in blood : **AMU 1986, 94**

A. Insulin treatment of diabetic patients
B. Inactivation of hormone sensitive lipase of adipose tissues
C. Prolonged fasting and uncontrolled diabetes mellitus
D. Excessive intake of high protein diet

Ans. **45. D** **46. C** **47. C** **48. D** **49. C** **50. B**
51. D **52. C** **53. C**

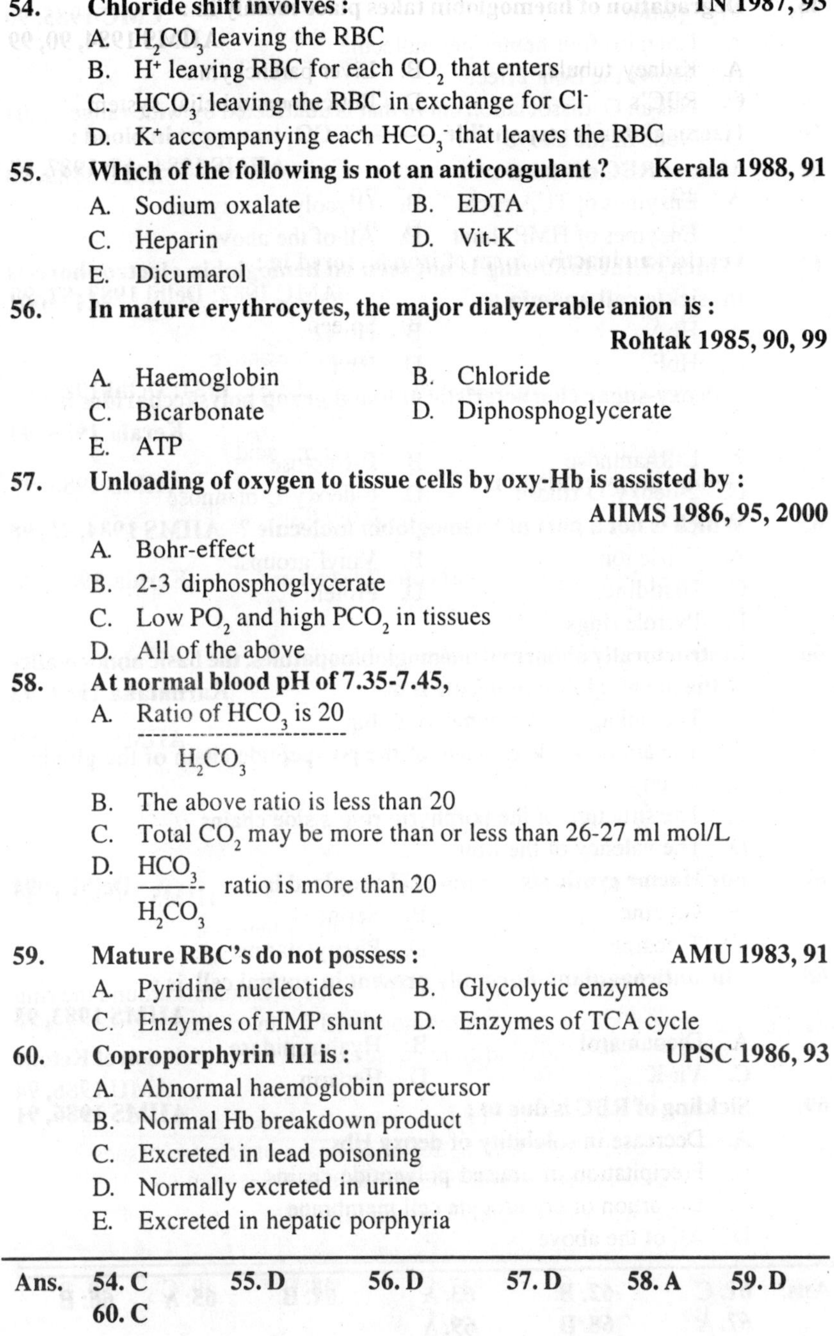

54. Chloride shift involves : **TN 1987, 93**

A. H_2CO_3 leaving the RBC

B. H^+ leaving RBC for each CO_2 that enters

C. HCO_3^- leaving the RBC in exchange for Cl^-

D. K^+ accompanying each HCO_3^- that leaves the RBC

55. Which of the following is not an anticoagulant ? **Kerala 1988, 91**

A. Sodium oxalate B. EDTA

C. Heparin D. Vit-K

E. Dicumarol

56. In mature erythrocytes, the major dialyzerable anion is : **Rohtak 1985, 90, 99**

A. Haemoglobin B. Chloride

C. Bicarbonate D. Diphosphoglycerate

E. ATP

57. Unloading of oxygen to tissue cells by oxy-Hb is assisted by : **AIIMS 1986, 95, 2000**

A. Bohr-effect

B. 2-3 diphosphoglycerate

C. Low PO_2 and high PCO_2 in tissues

D. All of the above

58. At normal blood pH of 7.35-7.45,

A. Ratio of $\frac{HCO_3}{H_2CO_3}$ is 20

B. The above ratio is less than 20

C. Total CO_2 may be more than or less than 26-27 ml mol/L

D. $\frac{HCO_3}{H_2CO_3}$ ratio is more than 20

59. Mature RBC's do not possess : **AMU 1983, 91**

A. Pyridine nucleotides B. Glycolytic enzymes

C. Enzymes of HMP shunt D. Enzymes of TCA cycle

60. Coproporphyrin III is : **UPSC 1986, 93**

A. Abnormal haemoglobin precursor

B. Normal Hb breakdown product

C. Excreted in lead poisoning

D. Normally excreted in urine

E. Excreted in hepatic porphyria

Ans. **54. C** **55. D** **56. D** **57. D** **58. A** **59. D** **60. C**

61. **Myoglobin :** **CMC 1985, 90**
A. Contains four hemes per molecule
B. Shows the Bohr effect
C. Has an O_2 dissociation curve that is unaffected by wide range of pH
D. None of the above

62. **Mature RBC contains :** **AMU 1989, 93**
A. Enzymes of TCA cycle B. Glycolytic enzymes
C. Enzymes of HMP shunt D. All of the above

63. **Which of the following is not seen on hemoglobin electrophoresis in sickle cell anemia :** **AI 2001**
A. HbA B. HbA2
C. HbF D. HbS

64. **A deoxy-sugar characteristic of blood group polysaccharides is :** **Kerala 1988, 93**
A. L-Rhamnose B. L-fructose
C. 2-deoxy-D-ribose D. 6-deoxy-L-mannose

65. **Which is not a part of haemoglobin molecule ?** **AIIMS 1984, 85, 98**
A. Ferric ion B. Vinyl groups
C. Histidine D. Protein
E. Pyrrole rings

66. **In structurally abnormal haemoglobinopathies, the basic abnormality of the haemoglobin molecule is in :** **Karnataka 1987, 93**
A. The linkage of the heme to globin
B. The amino acid sequence of the polypeptide chain of the globin moiety
C. The structure of the porphyrin ring's side chains
D. The valency of the iron

67. **For Haeme synthesis, amino acid required is :** **Delhi 1994**
A. Glycine B. Serine
C. Tyrosine D. Phenylalanine

68. **The anticoagulant, normally present in animal cell is :** **AIIMS 1983, 95**
A. Dicoumarol B. Hyaluronidase
C. Vit-K D. Heparin

69. **Sickling of RBC is due to :** **AIIMS 1986, 91**
A. Decrease in solubility of deoxy Hbs
B. Precipitation of unused polyeptide chains
C. Distortion of erythrocyte cell membrane
D. All of the above

Ans. **61. C** **62. B** **63. A** **64. B** **65. A** **66. B**
67. A **68. D** **69. A**

70. Increased serum levels of bilirubin diglucoronide are seen in : Delhi 2001

A. Pre-hepatic jaundice
B. Obstructive jaundice
C. Criggler Najjar syndrome
D. Infective hepatitis

71. Half of the buffer capacity of blood is because of : AMC 1987, 92

A. HCO_3^- B. Protein
C. Hemoglobin D. All of the above

72. The enzyme which keeps the iron of hemoglobin in ferrous form is : DNB 1989, 90

A. Glucokinase B. Glutathione reductase
C. Enolase D. Aldolase

73. Blood group antigens belong to the class—— : AP 1988, 91

A. Conjugated proteins
B. Unconjugated proteins
C. Simple proteins
D. Hemoglobin binding proteins

74. In normal adult the quantity of haemoglobin catalysed is : AIIMS 1987, 93

A. 2 g B. 4 g
C. 8 g D. 16 g

75. Protein present in haemoglobin has the structure known as : AIIMS 1984, 98

A. Primary B. Secondary
C. Tertiary D. Quarternary

76. Which of the following is recognized human blood coagulation factor : PGI 1982, 88, 97

A. Glutathione
B. Antihemophilic factor-A
C. N-acetyl D-galactosamine
D. D-glucoronic acid

77. All four amino terminal group of Hemoglobin can bind one molecule of : AIIMS 1985, 95

A. H^+ B. CO_2
C. CO D. Diphosphoglycerate

78. Liver does not produce : AIIMS 1983; AI 1989, 95

A. Albumin B. Gamma globulin
C. Fibrinogen D. Prothrombin

Ans. **70. B** **71. A** **72. B** **73. A** **74. C** **75. B**
76. B **77. B** **78. B**

79. APT test is used for : **PGI 1998**

A. Albumin B. Foetal Hb
C. Bence Jones proteins D. Myoglobin

80. Haemoglobin is a good buffer because of : **TNPSC 2000**

A. Histidine residue B. Protein nature
C. Acidic nature D. Iron molecule

81. Myoglobin : **TNPSC 2000**

A. Shows the Bohr effect
B. Has an oxygen dissociation curve that is unaffected over a wide range
C. Is an auxiliary system for oxygen transport in the blood
D. Contains four hemes per molecule

82. Highest binding of iron in plasma is seen with : **AI-2001**

A. Transferrin B. Ferritin
C. Hemoglobin D. Ceruloplasmin

83. Which of the following can be a homologous substitution for valine in hemoglobin? **AI 2004**

A. Isoleucine B. Glutamic acid
C. Phenylalanine D. Lysine

84. HbS has defect in amino acid position : **PGI 1984, TN 1991**

A. 4 B. 6
C. 11 D. 12

85. White hair are due to : **AP 1989, 96**

A. Deficiency of melanin
B. High content of iron
C. Increased proportion of Ca and PO_4
D. Decreased proportion of calcium carbonate and phosphate

86. Hemoglobin electrophoresis is based on : **AIIMS 2007**

A. Molecular weight
B. Charge
C. Solubility
D. Calorimetric properties

87. Within the RBC, hypoxia stimulates glycolysis by which of the following regulating pathways ? **AI 2007**

A. Hypoxia stimulates pyruvate dehydrogenase by increased 2, 3 DPG
B. Hypoxia inhibits hexokinase
C. Hypoxia stimulates release of all Glycolytic enzymes from Band 3 on RBC membrane
D. Activation of the regulatory enzymes by high pH

Ans. **79. B** **80. A** **81. D** **82. A** **83. B** **84. B**
85. C **86. B** **87. C**

88. **Gamma carboxylation of glutamic acid in clotting factors-II, VII and protein-C is dependent on :** **AI 2008**

A. Vitamin-K B. Vitamin-C
C. Vitamin-A D. Vitamin-E

89. **Thrombin activity is inhibited by :** **AI 2008**

A. Chymotrypsin B. Heparin cofactor-II
C. Alpha 2 antitrypsin D. Alpha 2 macroglobulin

Ans. **88. A** **89. B**

EXPLANATIONS OF BIOCHEMICAL ASPECTS

1. Ans. — A **Shift of oxyhemoglobin curve to the right**

* **Morgan's Anaesthesia writes :**

— **"Smoking should be discontinued for at least 6-8 weeks before the operation to decrease secretions and to reduce pulmonary complications. Cigarette smoking increases mucus production and decreases clearance. Both gaseous and particulate phase of cigarette smoke can deplete glutathione and vitamin-C and may promote oxidative injury to tissues.**

Carbon monoxide increaes carboxy-hemoglobin levels, while breakdown products of nitric oxide and nitrogendioxide can increase methemoglobin levels. Cessation of smoking for as little as 24 hours therefore has theoretically beneficial effects on oxygen carrying capacity of hemoglobin, because it decreases carboxyhemoglobin level, this shifts the O2 dissociation curve to the right."

* **Know that :**

* **Ciggaarette smoking causes increased production of carbon monoxide which has higher affinity for haemoglobin than O2. This leads to production of carboxyhemoglobin, in cigarette smokers as much as 20% of Hb is in the form of carboxyhemoglobin. This has two consequences :**

- **20% of Hb is not available for binding O2.**
- **the Hb-dissociation curve is shifted to left (this leads to decreased oxygen release in tissues)**

2. Ans. — B **Glutamic acid :**

* **Although substitution of one amino acid for another (due to single base changes in structural genes) are capable of inducing unacceptable mutations, (e.g. Hemoglobin produced by substitution of valine for glutamic acid at position 6 on β chain.** ***Some mutation have no apparent effect.***

* **'It has been shown that the codon for valine at position 67 of the β chain is not identical in all persons who posses a normally functional β chain of Hb' - *Harper*.**

This means that normally functional haemoglobin may have different amino acid at position 67 of β chains in place of valine.

- **When glutamic acid is present at position 67 in place of valine : Hb Milwaukee (Functionally normal)**
- **When asparitic acid is present at position 67 in place of valine : Hb Bristol (Functionally normal)**

Homozygous Substitution Amino Acids in place or Valine at position 67 of β chain	*Functionally normal Haemo-with other & globin type*
Glutamic acid	**Hb Milwaukee**
Aspartic acid	**Hb Bristol**
Alanine	**Hb Sydney**

Thus any of the above amino acids, can be a homologous substitution for valine with no apparent effect and result in functionally normal haemoglobin.

3. Ans.— A. Cystine

4. Ans.— C. Ferrous ions only

Iron in haemoglobin exists as ferrous ions only; its oxidation to ferric ion generates methaemoglobin which is ineffective as oxygen transporter.

5. Ans.— B. Beta chain of globin

The sickle cell mutation is replacement of a polar amino acid (glutamate) by a nonpolar amino acid (valine) in the beta chain of haemoglobin.

6. Ans.— C. Ecxess of bile salts in the urine

7. Ans.— C. 28

8. Ans.— A. Amino acids are excreted and iron preserved

9. Ans.— B. Effect of pCO2 on oxyhemoglobin

10. Ans.— A. HCO_3^- leaving the RBC in exchange for Cl^-

11. Ans.— B. Enzymes of TCA cycle

Tricarboxylic acid (TCA) cycle occurs in mitochondria, which are not present in mature RBCs. Therefore, enzymes of TCA cycle are not present in erythrocytes.

12. Ans.— B. Heparin
13. Ans.— D. Ferric ions
14. Ans.— B. HDL
15. Ans.— D. Sulphated D-Glucosamine and D-Glucuronic acid
16. Ans.— C. Hill's index-1
17. Ans.— B. Hydrophobic pockets
18. Ans.— A. O_2Hb + K hemoglobinate
19. Ans.— A. Beta - 6 glutamate by valine
20. Ans.— D. Transferrin
21. Ans.— C. Hb→Heme→Biliverdin→Bilirubin → Urobilinogen
22. Ans.— C. Methaemoglobin, Chloroform
23. Ans.— B. 16,800
24. Ans.— C. Dirty green
25. Ans.— D. Any of the above
26. Ans.— D. Methylene
27. Ans.— D. Green
28. Ans.— D. A very similar subunit of amino acid sequence
29. Ans.— A. V
30. Ans.— A. Dicoumarol
31. Ans.— D. Gamma
32. Ans.— C. Three lobed
33. Ans.— A. Increased CO2 tension
34. Ans.— B. H+
35. Ans.— C. IV
36. Ans.— A. Salt bridges are numerous
37. Ans.— C. XIII
38. Ans.— C. 6
39. Ans.— B. Porphyrin
40. Ans.— B. 0.8-1.1
41. Ans.— D. None of the above
42. Ans.— B. Beta chain
43. Ans.— A. Urokinase
44. Ans.— C. 7.4
    Normal blood pH lies within the range of 7.35 to 7.45
45. Ans.— D. Reticuloendothelial system
46. Ans.— C. 90
47. Ans.— C. Liver
48. Ans.— D. Ascorbic acid
49. Ans.— C. 0.9-1.0
50. Ans.— B. After splenectomy

51. Ans. — D. Protoporphyrin-IX

Haem in haemoglobin has 4 pyrrole rings, joined cavalently. The substituent groups in pyrrole rings are methyl (M), vinyl (V) and propionate (P), as shown in the Fig. below.

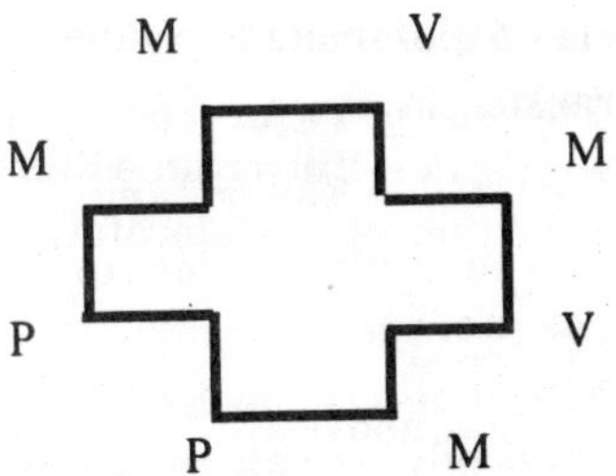

This cyclic structure is termed protoporphyri-IX. Chelation of iron at center of protoporphyrin yields haeme.

52. Ans. — C. Differs from coproporphyrin-III in the substituents around the ring

Uroporphyrinogen-III (not uropor-phyrinogen-I) is an intermediate in biosynthesis of haem (Option A). Conversion of uroporphyrinogen-III to uroporphyrinogen-I occurs *spontaneously* upon exposure to light; it does not require mediation of an oxidase (Option D).

Uroporphyrinogen-III contain a (cyclic) tetrapyrrole ring (Option B)

Different substituent groups a coproporphyrinogen and uropor-phyrinogen are shown in the Fig. below

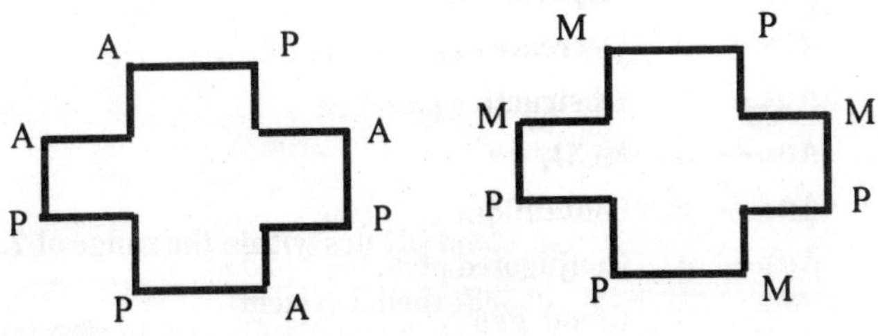

A = Acetate

P = Propimates

M = Methyl

53. Ans.— C. Prolonged fasting and uncontrolled diabetes mellitus

54. Ans.— C. HCO_3^- leaving the RBC in exchange for Cl^-

55. Ans.— D. Vit K

56. Ans.— D. Diphosphoglycerate

57. Ans.— D. All of the above

58. Ans.— A. Ratio of $\frac{HCO_3}{H_2CO_3}$ is 20

59. Ans.— D. Enzymes of TCA cycle

60. Ans.— C. Excreted in lead poisoning

61. Ans.— C. Has an O_2 dissociation curve that is unaffected by wide range of pH

Myoglobin contains a single haem molecule attached non-covalently to a polypeptide chain. It does not show Bohr's effect, i.e., unloading of oxygen in response to fall in pH or increased pCO2. Its oxygen dissociation curve, therefore, remains unaffected over a wide range of pH.

Haemoglobin is an oligomeric protein, and therefore has quaternary structure.

62. Ans.— B. Glycolytic enzymes

63. Ans.— A. HbA

64. Ans.— B. L-fructose

65. Ans.— A. Ferric ion

66. Ans.— B. The amino acid sequence of the polypeptide chain of the globin moiety

67. Ans.— A. Glycine

68. Ans.— D. Heparin

69. Ans.— A. Decrease in solubility of deoxy Hbs

70. Ans.— B. Obstructive jaundice

71. Ans.— A. HCO_3^-

72. Ans.— B. Glutathione reductase

73. Ans.— A. Conjugated proteins

Blood group antigens consist of saccharides linked covalently with proteins. Such structures having "protein + non-protein portions, linked covalently" are called conjugated proteins.

74. Ans.— C. 8 g

75. Ans.— B. **Secondary**

Proteins consisting of two, three or more polypeptide chains are called oligomeric proteins. Spatial relationship of different polypeptide subunits with one another is called quaternary structure.

76. Ans.— B. **Antihemophilic factor-A**

77. Ans.— B. **CO_2**

78. Ans.— B. **Gamma globulin**

79. Ans.— B. **Foetal Hb**

80. Ans.— A. **Histidine residue**

Histidine has an ionizable group present in the imidazole group of its side chains. The pK' value of imidazole being 6.0, the chains can act as buffer in the pH range of 6.0±1 which is very close to physiologic pH. Hence histidine R group is capable of providing buffering action at the physiologic pH.

81. Ans.— D. **Contains four hemes per molecule**

82. Ans.— A. **Transferrin**

83. Ans.— B. **Glutamic acid**

If valine at position 67 of the β chain of HbA is replaced by any of the following amino acids would result in no change in the function of Hb:

- **Alanine (Hb Sydney)**
- **Aspartatem (Hb Bristol) : AAG**
- **Glutamate (Hb Milwaukee)**

84. Ans.— B. **6**

85. Ans.— C. **Increased proportion of Ca and PO_4**

86. Ans.— B **Charge**

Each of the major hemglobin types has an electrical charge of a different degree, so the most useful method for separating and measuring normal and abnormal hemoglobins is electrophoresis.

87. Ans.— C **Hypoxia stimulates release of all Glycolytic enzymes from Band 3 on RBC membrane**

Hypoxia causes Deoxygenation of Haemoglobin and increases band 3 Tyrosine Phosphorylation. This stimulates the releasing of all Glycolytic Enzymes from Band 3 on the RBC membrane thereby stimulating Glycolysis.

88. Ans. — A Vitamin-K

Vitamin-K is required for the conversion of several clotting factors and prothrombin precursors to the active state. The mechanism of this action has been most clearly delineated for prothrombin.

89. Ans. — B Heparin cofactor-II

Thrombin activity is inhibited by :

1. **Heparin cofactor-II**
2. **Alpha-1 antitrypsin and**
3. **Antithrombin-III**

Direct thrombin inhibitors such as bivalirudin, lepirudin, and argatroban are a new class of anticoagulants.

PHYSIOLOGICAL ASPECTS

IMPORTANT TEXT FOR PHYSIOLOGICAL ASPECTS

METABOLIC CHANGES IN SHOCK

Plasma/blood	Cells	Urine
↑ Glucose	↓ O2 consumption	↑ Ketones
↓ pH	↓ Glucose oxidation	↑ N2
↑ Lactate	Glycogen depletion	
↑ FFA	Mobilization of fat	
↑ Glycerol	Depletion of ATP	
↑ NPN	↓ Membrane Potential	
	↑ Gluconeogenosis	

* In hypovolemic shock, grading is also done by fall in BP—— mild (upto ↓ 20%), moderate (upto ↓ 40%) and severe (↓ above 40%).
* Diisopropyl fluorophosphate is called nerve gas.
* Acidosis means fall of pH below 7.35 and alkalosis pH above 7.45.
* Tm of important substances :

  Glucose - 320 mg/min, Urate - 15 mg/min,

  Hemoglobin - 1.2 mg/min, plasma protein 25-30 mg/min,

  Amino acid - 1.4 mg/min
* Total amount of fluid filtered by both, kidneys per min is called **'Tubular Load'**
* Normal glomerular pressure is 60 mm Hg
* Normal capsular pressure in 18 mm Hg
* Normal colloid osmotic pressure is 32 mmHg
* Normal filtration pressure is 10 mmHg

GAS CONTENT OF BLOOD

Gas	*ml/dl of Blood Containing 15g of Hemoglobin*			
	Arterial Blood (PO_2 95 mm Hg; PCO_2 40 mm Hg; Hb 97% Saturated)		Venous Blood (PO_2 40 mm Hg; PCO_2 46 mm Hg; Hb75% Saturated)	
	Dissolved	*Combined*	*Dissolved*	*Combined*
O_2	0.29	19.5	0.12	15.1
CO_2	2.62	46.4	2.98	49.7
N_2	0.98	0	0.98	0

FATE OF CO_2 IN BLOOD

In plasma

1. Dissolved
2. Formation of carbamino compounds with plasma protein
3. Hydration, H^+ buffered, HCO_3^- in plasma

In red blood cells

1. Dissolved
2. Formation of carbamino-Hb
3. Hydration, H^+ buffered, 70% of HCO_3^- diffuses into plasma
4. Cl^- shifts into cells; mOsm/liter in cells increases

MCQ'S FOR PHYSIOLOGICAL ASPECTS

1. **Which of the following favours filtration in the arteriolar end of the capillary bed ? AIIMS 2006**
   A. Increased oncotic pressure in the capillaries
   B. Decreased hydrostatic pressure in capillaries
   C. Decreased oncotic pressure in capillaries
   D. Increased oncotic pressure in the interstitium
2. **Arterial blood gas of a 5 year old child done at sea level gives the following results : pH 7.41, PaO_2 100 mmHg, and $PaCO_2$ to mm Hg. This child is being ventilated with 80% oxygen. What is the (A-a) PO_2: AIIMS-2005**
   A. 570.4 mm Hg B. 520.4 mm Hg
   C. 470.4 mm Hg D. 420.4 mm Hg
3. **Which of the following situation will lead to increased viscosity of blood : AIIMS-2005**
   A. Fasting state B. Hypoglycemia
   C. Multiple myeloma D. Amyloidogenesis
4. **The velocity of blood is maximum in the : AIIMS-2005**
   A. Large veins B. Small veins
   C. Venules D. Capillaries
5. **Which of the following conditions lead to tissue hypoxia without alteration of oxygen content of blood ? AIIMS-2005**
   A. CO poisoning B. Met Hb
   C. Cyanide poisoning D. Respiratory acidosis
6. **Vasoconstriction is exhibited by all except : AMC 1984**
   A. Valsalva manoeuvre B. Asphyxia
   C. Haemorrhage D. Lying down

Directions for Questions (below)(Ques7 to 10) for each type of blood vessel listed below, choose the characteristic with which it is usually associated : AIIMS 1982, 89

A. Arteries B. Arterioles
C. Capillaries D. Venules
E. Veins

Ans. 1. C 2. D 3. C 4. A 5. C 6. D

7. **Slowest pulmonary compliance**
8. **Lowest hydrostatic pressure**
9. **Least resistance to blood flow**
10. **Largest surface area**
11. **Blood flow in carotid body in ml/100g of tissue** **AMU 1987, 97**

A. 500 B. 1000
C. 2000 D. 4000

12. **Which of the following is most fatal complication of increased barometric pressure :** **AMC 1983, 93**

A. Oxygen toxicity B. Nitrogen narcosis
C. Air embolism D. Decompensation sickness

13. **Administration of oxygen rich gas mixtures is of value in all except :** **PGI 1982, 98**

A. Histotoxic hypoxia B. Stagnant hypoxia
C. Anemic hypoxia D. Hypoxic hypoxia

14. **Carbon monoxide reacts with hemoglobin to form:** **UPSC 1985, 98**

A. Carboxy hemoglobin
B. Reduced hemoglobin
C. Cyanmethemoglobin
D. Any of the above

15. **Hemoglobin has ——— times affinity for carbon monoxide than oxygen :** **AMC 1985, 95**

A. 50 B. 100
C. 210 D. 320

16. **The most common form of hypoxia is :** **AIIMS 1996**

A. Hypoxic B. Stagnant
C. Anemic D. Histotoxic

17. **Causes of hypoxic hypoxia include all except :** **Rohtak 1988, 93**

A. Kyphoscoliosis B. Emphysema
C. Pulmonary fibrosis D. Carbon monoxide poisoning

18. **The carotid bodies have the following features, except :** **PGI 1980, 90**

A. Have blood flow rate similar to that of brain.
B. More influenced by arterial PO_2 than by arterial oxygen content.
C. Stimulated by a rise in blood hydrogen ion concentration.
D. Along with aortic bodies are wholly responsible for stimulation of ventilation in response to hypoxia.

Ans.	7. C	8. E	9. C	10. C	11. C	12. C
	13. A	14. A	15. C	16. A	17. D	18. A

19. All of the following statements about the monocytes are true except: **Manipal 1995, 98**

A. They originate from precursors in the bone marrow
B. They can ingest dead granulocytes
C. They may migrate from the blood into the tissues
D. They can manufacture immunoglobulins

20. Oxygen dissociation curve is sigmoid in shape because of : **JIPMER 1986, 99**

A. Shifting affinity for oxygen
B. Shifting affinity for CO_2
C. Blood pH
D. All of the above

21. Direct Fick method of measuring cardiac output requires estimation of : **DNB 1989, 96**

A. O_2 content of arterial blood
B. O_2 consumption per unit time
C. Arteriovenous O_2 difference
D. O_2 content of blood from right ventricle

22. A shift of the oxygen dissociation curve of blood to the right is a feature not found : **PGI 1986, 99**

A. In pulmonary capillaries
B. With rise in temperature
C. When foetal blood is replaced by adult blood
D. In all of the above

23. Select the statement which is best characterises lymph capillaries: **Rohtak 1986, 99**

A. Have smaller diameter than blood capillaries
B. Less permeable than blood capillaries
C. Have no endothelial lining
D. Have a discontinuous basement membrane

24. What best characterises the sinusoids ? **AMU 1986, 99**

A. Have smaller diameter than lymph capillaries
B. Are not found in skeletal muscle
C. Have a continuous endothelial lining
D. Have a continuous basement membrane

25. A substance on I.V. injection was found to be distributed through thirty percent of body water. It probably : **DNB 1988, 98**

A. Did not pass freely through blood capillaries
B. Was distributed evenly throughout body water
C. Did not enter cells of body
D. Was excluded from CSF

Ans. **19. D** **20. A** **21. D** **22. A** **23. D** **24. B** **25. C**

26. **To estimate cardiac output by dye-dilution technique, dye concentration is measured in : DNB 1989, 94**
   A. Sample from peripheral artery
   B. Sample from right atrium
   C. Sample from aorta
   D. Sample from pulmonary artery continuously

Match the following(Ques. 27 to 33) : AIIMS 1986, 96
   A. Anaemic anoxia B. Anoxic anoxia
   C. Histotoxic anoxia D. Stagnant anoxia

27. **Venous pO_2 higher than normal:**
28. **Mercury poisoning of respiratory enzymes :**
29. **Thromboembolism occluding a leg vein**
30. **Breathing atmospheric air at high altitude :**
31. **Drowning :**
32. **Excessive blood loss :**
33. **Carbon monoxide poisoning of Hb :**
34. **Following are increased during exercise except : AP 1997, 99**
   A. Cardiac output
   B. Venous rectum
   C. Coronary blood flow
   D. Peripheral vascular resistance
35. **The prime regulator of blood flow through exercising muscles is: AIIMS 1983, 87**
   A. Venous tone
   B. Sympathetic control
   C. Vasodilator metabolites
   D. Parasympathetic control
36. **The law relating distending pressure and tension in a blood vessels wall is called : AIIMS 1985, 98**
   A. Frank Starling's law B. Einthoven's law
   C. Law of Laplace D. Mary's law
37. **Vascular distensibility is least for the following vascular segment: DNB 1989, 95**
   A. Pulmonary artery B. Systemic artery
   C. Systemic vein D. Pulmonary vein

Ans.	**26. A**	**27. D**	**28. C**	**29. D**	**30. B**	**31. B**
	32. A	**33. A**	**34. D**	**35. C**	**36. C**	**37. B**

38. At a constant pressure gradient across the ends of a vessel, the laminar flow through the vessel is proportional to :

AIIMS 1993, 98

A. Square of the radius (R)
B. $1/R_2$
C. $1/R_4$
D. R_4

39. Turbulant blood flow is produced by : **Delhi 1988, 99**

A. Decreased velocity of circulation
B. Decreased cardiac output
C. Decreased haematocrit
D. All of the above

40. Factors which increase the hardness of arterial walls :

AMC 1984, 98

A. Decrease in the velocity of arterial pulse
B. Increase in peripheral resistance
C. Raised systolic blood pressure
D. Raised diastolic blood pressure

41. Venoconstriction is exhibited by following except :

Delhi 1990, 91

A. Valsalva manoeuvre
B. Asphyxia
C. Haemorrhage
D. Lying down
E. Carotid artery occlusion

42. Blood flow is largely regulated by local metabolic effects in :

AI 1991

A. Kidney B. Muscle
C. Bone D. Skin

43. The arterial pulse pressure in the femoral artery is normally :

PGI 1980,99

A. Less than the pulse pressure in the upper aorta
B. Less than 20 mmHg
C. Greater than the pulse pressure in the upper aorta
D. Equal to the pulse pressure in the upper aorta

44. The most dializable anion in RBC is : **Bihar 1998, 99**

A. Hemoglobin B. Cl^-
C. HCO_3^- D. PO_4^{3-}

Ans. **38. D** **39. C** **40. C** **41. D** **42. B** **43. C** **44. C**

45. What is the correct sequence of the following events that lead to regulation of blood volume by the kidney when the blood volume is raised ? **CSE 1997**

1. Increase in GFR and urine output
2. Increase in arterial blood pressure
3. Increase in cardiac output
4. Decrease in blood volume

Select the correct answer using the codes given below:

A. 3,1,2,4 B. 1,3,2,4
C. 3,2,1,4 D. 1,2,3,4

46. The pressure at one end of an artery is 60 mm Hg, the pressure at the other end of the artery is 20 mm Hg, and the flow through the artery of 200 ml/min. What is the resistance of the artery expressed in the above units ? **PGI 1982, 99**

A. 0.05 B. 0.1
C. 0.2 D. 0.4

47. Oncotic pressure is measured by : **Rajasthan 1995, 96**

A. Osmal B. Joule
C. mm of Hg D. Kg/m^2

48. Pulse pressure is lowest in : **AIIMS 1993, 98**

A. Capillaries B. Arterioles
C. Radial artery D. Femoral artery

49. Which causes a left shift of the oxygen dissociation curve :
AI 1993, Delhi 1988, 97; PGI 2000

A. ↓ Diphosphoglycerate
B. ↑ 2,3 DPG
C. ↓ Lactate
D. ↑ Lactate

50. A Right sided shift of the oxygen dissociation curve is caused by :
AI 1993, Delhi 1987, 97

A. ↓ 2, 3DPG B. Hyperthermia
C. Hypothermia D. Low Altitudes

51. In cellular hypoxia, following are seen except :
Delhi 1992, 99

A. Cellular swelling B. Loss of ATP
C. Extrusion of Na D. None of the above

52. Autoregulation of blood flow is carried out by :
AP 1991, JIPMER 1992

A. Muscles B. Potassium
C. Substance P D. Kinins

Ans. **45. B** **46. C** **47. A** **48. A** **49. C** **50. B**
51. C **52. B**

53. Shift in Oxygen dissociation curve to the right is caused by : JIPMER 1990, 92

A. Raised 2-3 DPG B. Raised pH
C. Raised PO2 D. Low PCO2

54. 'J' receptors stimulation causes : AIIMS 1992, 99

A. Tachycardia B. Hypertension
C. Apnoea D. Tachynoea

55. The pressure required to occlude blood flow with a tourniquet exceeds systolic pressure by : JIPMER 1992, 98

A. 4 mm Hg
B. 25-50 mm Hg
C. Twice systolic pressure
D. None of the above

56. The amount of O_2 in blood is determined by the : AMC 1985,99

A. Amount of dissolved O_2
B. Amount of hemoglobin in blood
C. Affinity of hemoglobin for oxygen
D. All of the above

57. In arterial blood, hemoglobin which is satured with O_2 is : AMU 1987, 99

A. 100% B. 97%
C. 87% D. 75%

58. Which of the following is true about composition of venous blood: AIIMS 1982, 99

	PO_2 (mmHg)	PCO_2 (mmHg)	Hb saturated (%)
A.	95	40	75
B.	40	40	75
C.	40	46	75
D.	46	40	75

59. The presence of hemoglobin increase the oxygen carrying capacity of the blood : Delhi 1982, 99

A. 30 fold B. 50 fold
C. 70 fold D. 100 fold

60. Heart receives about____ % of cardiac output : UPSC 1983, 93

A. 1 B. 2
C. 5 D. 10

61. The commonest cause of sustained diastolic hypertension is : UPSC 1984, 94

A. Unknown B. Conn's syndrome
C. Renal disease D. Phaeochromocytoma

Ans. 53. A 54. D 55. B 56. D 57. B 58. C
59. C 60. C 61. A

62. Hepatic venous pressure is : Delhi 1983, 93

A. 22 mmHg in man B. 3 mmHg in man
C. 5 mmHg in man D. 10 mmHg in man

63. Hepatic blood flow is : AMC 1987, 98

A. 500 ml/min B. 800 ml/min
C. 1200 ml/min D. 1500 ml/min

64. Blood flow reaching the liver via portal versus hepatic artery is: AMU 1986, 98

A. 2 : 1 B. 3 : 1
C. 4 : 1 D. 6 : 1

65. The most important response to the stimulation of beta adrenergic receptors is : AIIMS 1980, 99

A. Cerebral vasodilation
B. Splanchnic vasoconstriction
C. Decreased blood sugar
D. Increased cardiac activity

66. Major part of total peripheral resistance is : DNB 1989, 95

A. Medium and small arteries
B. Venules
C. Capillaries
D. Arterioles

67. Which of the following has the maximum oxygen consumption (ml/min) : AMC 1982, 89

A. Brain B. Skeletal muscle
C. Heart muscle D. Kidneys

68. A-V oxygen difference is maximum in : AMU 1986, 89

A. Skeletal muscle B. Brain
C. Heart muscle D. Liver

69. After liver and kidneys, the blood flow is maximum in : TN 1986,87, 99

A. Brain B. Skeletal muscle
C. Skin D. Heart muscle

70. Which of the following shows the maximum absolute resistance : AMU 1986, 99

A. Skin B. Brain
C. Heart D. Liver

71. In capillaries, blood flow at the rate of —— cm/sec: Delhi 1996, 98

A. 0.007 B. 0.07
C. 0.15 D. 1.0

Ans. 62. C 63. A 64. A 65. D 66. D 67. B
68. C 69. B 70. C 71. B

72. **Which of the following organ has the maximum weight :** **AMC 1985, 95**
A. Liver B. Kidneys
C. Brain D. Heart

73. **Blood flow in ml/100g/min is maximum in :** **Delhi 1980, 99**
A. Kidneys B. Liver
C. Heart D. Skin

74. **Blood pressure is not reliable in :** **Rohtak 1985, 99**
A. Coarctation of aorta B. Pulmonary stenosis
C. Atrial fibrillation D. Polyarteritis nodosa

75. **Plasma CO2 content is :** **UPSC 1989, 99**
A. 10-12 mm/L B. 15-18 mm/L
C. 25-28 mm/L D. 32-35 mm/L

76. **The average normal arm to tongue circulation time is :** **AMU 1984, 94**
A. 5 sec B. 10 sec
C. 15 sec D. 30 sec

77. **Normal A-V O_2 difference at rest is :** **UPSC 1980, 94**
A. 2.1 ml B. 3.4 ml
C. 4.3 ml D. 5.6 ml

78. **Caliber of the arterioles is increased by following except :** **AMU 1985, 98**
A. Circulating angiotensin-II
B. Kinins
C. Increased PCO_2
D. Decreased pH

79. **"Axon reflex"—— the arteriole :** **AMU 1984, 95**
A. Dilate B. Constricts
C. A or B D. Does not affect

80. **On Poiseuille Hagen formula, the relationship is calculated between following except :** **AMU 1984, 96**
A. Flow in a long narrow tube
B. Viscosity of fluid
C. Radius of tube
D. pH of blood

81. **Dopamine is used in the treatment of shock because it is :** **AMC 1986, 89; AIIMS 1982, 83, 85**
A. Strongly ionotropic
B. Strongly chronotropic
C. Increased renal arterial blood flow
D. All of the above

Ans. **72. A** **73. A** **74. C** **75. C** **76. C** **77. C**
78. A **79. A** **80. D** **81. C**

82. Which of the following changes would tend to cause accumulation of fluid (edema) in the tissues : AIIMS 1985, 94

A. Increased precapillary vascular resistance
B. Decreased postcapillary vascular resistance
C. Increased plasma colloid osmotic pressure
D. Increased venous pressure

83. Which of the following change would probably occur as a result of two fold increase in the net filtration of fluid into the tissue : AIIMS 1984, 94

A. A marked increase in lymph flow rate
B. Approximately a two-fold increase in interstitial fluid volume
C. A decrease in interstitial fluid colloid osmotic pressure
D. a and b
E. a and c

W.84. Which of the following would not be expected to cause hypoxia : AIIMS 1984, 96

A. Hypoventilation
B. Abnormal ventilation to perfusion ratio
C. Diminished diffusing capacity for O_2
D. Excessive blood flow through venous to arterial shunt

85. Maximum surface area of circulating system is seen in : PGI 1985, 88

A. Arteries
B. Vein
C. Arterioles
D. Capillaries

86. Which of the following statements about erythropoietin is false? Manipal 1996

A. It is a glycoprotein
B. It has been isolated in the pure form
C. It is mainly produced by the bone marrow
D. It can be measured by radioimmunoassay

87. Following acute failure of the left ventricle of the heart in man, pulmonary edema generally begins to appear when left atrial pressure approaches : AIIMS 1980, 98

A. 7 mm Hg
B. 15 mm Hg
C. 20 mm Hg
D. 30 mm Hg

88. When a normal person suddenly changes from recumbant to standing posture : AIIMS 1981, 98

A. Blood pressure falls dramatically
B. Renin secretion is suppressed
C. Blood pools in the jugular vein
D. Heart rate increases

Ans. 82. D 83. E 84. NONE 85. D 86. C 87. D 88. D

89. **Vasovagal syncope is called :** **AIIMS 1985; Delhi 1986, 98**
A. Hypovolemic shock
B. Anaphylactic shock
C. Emotional shock
D. Septicemic shock

90. **Dilatation of capillaries may result due to :** **Delhi 1984, 89, 94**
A. 5-HT B. Norepinephrine
C. Low temperature D. Axon reflex

91. **Coronary blood flow stops during :** **Delhi 1989; UPSC 1991, 95**
A. Protodiastole
B. End of diastole
C. Isometric contraction
D. Isovolumetric contraction

92. **After haemorrhage, restoration of blood volume is due to :**
AIIMS 1985, 95
A. Arterial constriction
B. Shift of intracellular fluid to extracellular space
C. Venous return increases
D. Intravenous infusion

93. **Consider the following statements :** **CSE 1997, 99**
Complete compensation for acid-base disturbances within a short time is characteristic of regulation by:
1. Chemical buffers
2. Respiratory regulatory system
3. Renal regulatory system
Of these statements
A. 1,2 and 3 are correct
B. 2 and 3 are correct
C. 3 alone is correct
D. 1 alone is correct

94. **Which one of the following is the correct sequence in increasing order of their basal blood supply (ml/min/100g of tissue)?**
CSE 1998, 99
A. Heart, brain, kidney B. Brain, kidney, heart
C. Kidney, heart, brain D. Brain, heart, kidney

95. **Hypoxia is characterised by :** **AIIMS 1984, 85, 90**
A. Low arterial PO_2
B. Intense chemoreceptor response
C. Favourable response to 100% oxygen
D. All of the above

Ans. **89. C** **90. D** **91. D** **92. B** **93. D** **94. D**
95. D

96. **Which of the following statements is incorrect : AMU 1986,98**
A. Blood velocity in capillary is greater than large vein.
B. Total surface area of the capillary is much greater than large veins.
C. Reduced O_2 tension in the tissue tend to relax pre-capillary sphineter.
D. Increased sympathetic nervous stimulation would tend to constrict the small arterioles.

97. **Peripheral chemoreceptors are not stimulated in which type of hypoxia : AI 1995; AIIMS 1995**
A. Hypoxic hypoxia B. Anaemic hypoxia
C. Stagnent hypoxia D. Histotoxic hypoxia

98. **In cyanide poisoning, there is : Delhi 1995, 99**
A. ↓ Cellular respiration
B. Cyanosis
C. ↓ O_2 transport
D. All of the above

99. **The arteriovenous oxygen difference (ml/L) is minimum in the following organ : AI 1995, 99**
A. Skin B. Skeletal muscle
C. Kidneys D. Liver

100. **Difference of pulmonary microcirculation from systemic one is : AI 1995, 99**
A. Resistance low, pulsatile flow
B. Resistance low, capillary pressure low
C. Capillary pressure high, pulsatile flow
D. Resistance high, capillary pressure high

101. **During exercise, blood does not decrease in : AI 1995**
A. Cutaneous circulation
B. Hepatosplanchinic circulation
C. Coronary circulation
D. Renal circulation

102. **Oxygen affinity is increased by following except : AI 1995**
A. Alkalosis B. Hypopnea
C. Increased HbF D. Hyperthermia

103. **The amount of blood in capillaries is : Rajasthan 1990, 94**
A. 30-50 ml B. 500-600 ml
C. 2-2.5 Litres D. 4-4.5 Litres

Ans. 96. A 97. D 98. A 99. C 100. B 101. C
102. D 103. B

104. Which of the following would not be expected to occur during sternuous physical exercise : AIIMS 1987, 99

A. Large ↑ Pulm. blood flow
B. Large ↑ Pulm. Artery pressure
C. Large ↓ Pulm. vascular resistance
D. Pulm. capillary distension
E. Pulm. capillary recruitment

105. Splanchnic vessels and venules contain —— % of blood volume : AMC 1986, 87

A. 10-20 B. 20-30
C. 40-50 D. 60-70

106. If the baroreceptor reflexes are fully functional when upright posture is assumed : AIIMS 1980, 90

A. Blood vessels of arm will be vasodilated
B. Arterial pressure in foot maintained at 120/80 mmHg
C. Bradycardia
D. Cerebral blood flow will not change appreciably

107. In a person who stands suddenly from lying posture, there is : Delhi 1997, 99

A. Increased different discharge from IX nerve
B. Increased tone of capacitance veins
C. Decreased HR
D. None of the above

108. A substance which has a distribution of 30-35% in body water is injected intravenously. True statement is : Rajasthan 1995

A. Distributed evenly through body water
B. Does not pass freely through capillary water
C. Distributed in cells only
D. Does not enter the body cells

109. Autoregulation of blood flow is seen in: AIIMS 1999; JIPMER 2000

A. Cardiac muscle B. Splanchnic blood flow
C. Cerebrum D. Spleen

110. The cardiac output can be determined by all except: PGI 1999

A. Fick's principle B. V/Q ratio
C. Angiocardiography D. Thermodilution

Ans. **104. B** **105. B** **106. D** **107. B** **108. D** **109. C** **110. B**

111. True about blood flow in various organs is : **PGI 1999**
A. Liver>Kidney>brain>heart
B. Liver>brain>kidney>heart
C. Kidney>brain>heart>liver
D. Liver>heart>brain>kidney

112. Pressure on carotid sinus causes : **PGI 1999**
A. Reflex bradycardia B. Tachycardia
C. Brainbridge reflex D. ↑ BP

113. Consider the following statements regarding nitric oxide : **UPSC 2000**
1. It is synthesized from L. Arginine
2. It is a vasodilator
3. It modifies platelet neutrophil interaction
4. It modifies release of prostaglandins.

Which of the following statements are correct ?
A. 1, 2 and 3 B. 2, 3 and 4
C. 1, 3 and 4 D. 1, 2 and 4

114. Endothelium derived relaxing factor (EDRF) is : **JIPMER 2000**
A. Nitric oxide B. Thromboxane A_2
C. Bradykinin D. Angiotensin

115. In which of the following organs will the rate of blood flow change the least during exercise ? **TNPSC 1998**
A. Skin B. Brain
C. Intestine D. Heart

116. True about Nitric oxide is : **UP 2000**
A. Synthesized from arginine
B. Spontaneous production from NO_2
C. Vasoconstriction
D. Released from mitochondria

117. A 0.5 litre blood loss in 30 minutes will lead to : **AI-2001**
A. Increase in HR, decrease in BP
B. Slight increase in HR, normal BP
C. Decrease in HR and BP
D. Prominent increase in HR

118. Albumin contributes maximum to oncotic pressure because of its : **AI 2001**
A. High mol. wt. low concentration
B. Low mol .wt. low concentration
C. High mol. wt. high concentration
D. Low mol. wt. high concentration

Ans. **111. A** **112. A** **113. A** **114. A** **115. C** **116. A**
117. B **118. D**

119. Increased radius of resistance vessels lead to : **Delhi 2001**

A. Increased systolic blood pressure
B. Increased diastolic blood pressure
C. Increased rate of blood flow
D. None of the above

120. Velocity of blood in capillaries is : **Delhi 2001**

A. 0.1 mm/sec B. 1 mm/sec
C. 5 mm/sec D. 10 mm/sec

121. Cyanosis with normal arterial O_2 concentration cause : **DNB 2001**

A. Anaemic hypoxia B. Stagnant hypoxia
C. Histotoxic hypoxia D. Hypoxic hypoxia

122. Mechanism of restoration of blood volume in acute hemorrhage is by : **Kerala 2001**

A. Vasoconstriction
B. Redistribution of body fluids
C. Heart rate increase
D. Heart rate decrease

123. In hypercarbia, which of the following is seen : **AIIMS 2001**

A. Hypertension B. Bradycardia
C. Cold clammy skin D. Miosis

124. A low lander lands at an attitude of 6500 m with an atmospheric pressure of 347 mm, the partial pressure of 0_2 is : **AIIMS 2002**

A. 53 B. 63
C. 73 D. 83

125. True about closed homeostatic treatment is : **AIIMS 2002**

A. Value of controlled variable is compared to the reference value
B. Positive feedback stabilizes system
C. Negative feedback
D. Oscillates around set point

126. Albumin does not pass through the glomerulus because of the presence of : **Maharashtra -2000**

A. Proteoglycans B. Glycolipid
C. Phospholipid D. Carbohydrates

127. Structure with richest blood supply is : **CMC 2001**

A. Retina B. Renal cortex
C. Heart D. Carotid body

Ans. **119. C** **120. C** **121. A** **122. B** **123. A** **124. A**
125. B **126. A** **127. D**

128. **Maximum pressure drop occurs at the level of :** **A.P.-2002**
A. Capillaries B. Small arteries
C. Large arteries D. Veins

129. **One intern calculated the concentration of O_2 in blood as 0.0025 ml/ml of blood. Considering atmospheric pressure as 760 mm Hg, how much approx. O_2 tension could have been in the blood?** **AI 2004**
A. 40 mm Hg B. 60 mm Hg
C. 80 mm Hg D. 100 mm Hg

130. **The blood in the vessels normally does not clot because?** **AI 2004**
A. Vitamin-K antagonists are present in plasma
B. Thrombin has a positive feedback on plasminogen
C. Sodium citrate in plasma chelates calcium ions
D. Vascular endothelium is smooth and coated with glycocalyx

131. **In which of the following, a reduction in arterial oxygen tension occurs?** **AI 2005**
A. Anaemia B. CO poisoning
C. Moderate exercise D. Hypoventilation

132. **The vasodilatation produced by carbon dioxide is maximum in one of the following :** **AI 2005**
A. Kidney B. Brain
C. Liver D. Heart

133. **Distribution of blood flow is mainly regulated by the :** **AI 2005**
A. Arteries B. Arterioles
C. Capillaries D. Venules

134. **CO_2 is primarily transported in the arterial blood as :** **AI 2005**
A. Dissolved CO_2
B. Carbonic Acid
C. Carbamino-hemoglobin
D. Bicarbonate

135. **The normal plasma oncotic pressure is :** **Kerala 1997**
A. 10 mmHg B. 15 mmHg
C. 20 mmHg D. 30 mmHg

136. **All of the following increase the interstitial pressure except :** **Delhi 1996**
A. ↓ Capillary permeability
B. ↑ Capillary permeability
C. a+b
D. None of the above

Ans. **128. B** **129. D** **130. D** **131. D** **132. B** **133. B**
134. D **135. D** **136. A**

137. Blood volume is equal to : UPSC 1983

A. Plasma Volume x $\frac{100}{100-0.87 \text{ haematocrit}}$

B. Plasma Volume x $\frac{100-0.87 \text{ haematocrit}}{100}$

C. Plasma Volume ÷ $\frac{100}{100-0.87 \text{ haematocrit}}$

D. Plasma Volume ÷ $\frac{100-0.87 \text{ haematocrit}}{100}$

138. Blood flow is largely regulated by local metabolic effects in : AIIMS 1983

A. Skin B. Brain
C. Kidney D. Muscle

139. Velocity of blood is ——— times that of urine : AIIMS 1982

A. Same as of ECF
B. 10 times of urine
C. 5-6 times more that of water
D. 5-6 times less that of water

140. When a person changes position from standing to lying down leads to: AIIMS 2007

A. Heart rate increases and settles at a higher level
B. Venous return to the heart rises immediately
C. Cerebral blood flow becomes more than in the standing position and settles at a higher level
D. Decrease in blood flow to the lung apex

141. O_2 delivery to tissues depends on all/except : AIIMS 2007

A. Cardiac output
B. Type of fluid administered
C. Hemoglobin concentration
D. Affinity of hemoglobin for O_2

142. Lymph flow from the foot is : AI 2008

A. Increased when an individual rises from the supine to standing position
B. Increased by massaging the foot
C. Increased when capillary permeability is decreased
D. Decreased when the valves of the leg veins are incompetent

---

Ans. 137. A 138. D 139. C 140. B 141. B 142. B

143. Venous flow in the lower limb veins in the standing position depends upon all except : AIIMS 2008

A. Arterial blood pressure
B. Presence of deep facial planes
C. Compressin of calf muscles
D. Presence of perforators

144. Stuart Power factor is factor : UPSC 1984, 94

A. VIII B. IX
C. X D. XII

145. MCHC (g/dl) is : AIIMS 1983; Delhi 1989, 99

A. 7.5 B. 29
C. 34 D. 87

146. Neutropenia is seen in all except : AIIMS 1984, 92

A. Pernicious anaemia
B. Severe bacterial infection
C. Trauma
D. Bone marrow depression

147. The most suitable anticoagulant for ESR determination by Wintrobe's method is : UPSC 1983, 86, 96

A. Sodium citrate B. EDTA
C. Heparin D. Double oxalatation

148. What does facitilate the conversion of profibrinolysin to fibrinolysin : AIIMS 1987

A. Tissue enzymes B. Streptokinase
C. Urokinase D. All of the above

149. Haemoglobin first appears in : AMU 1985, 86, 97

A. Early normoblast B. Intermediate normoblast
C. Late normoblast D. Pronormoblast

150. Aggregation of platelets is inhibited by : Delhi 1984

A. Ca^{++} B. ADP
C. Thrombin D. None of the above

151. The life span of platelets is : UPSC 1984, 99

A. 4 days B. 9-12 days
C. 20-30 days D. 90 days

152. The cell membrane of human erythrocytes is more permeable to: AIIMS 1986, 97

A. Cl^+ than K^+ B. K^+ than Na^+
C. K^+ than urea D. Glucose than glycerol

Ans. 143. B 144. C 145. C 146. C 147. B 148. D
149. B 150. D 151. B 152. B

153. Thrombosthenin is : **AIIMS 1984, 86, 97**
A. Coagulation factor
B. Contractile protein
C. A thrombosis promoting protein
D. A protein regulating platelet producing

154. Christmas disease results to lack of which of the following factor of coagulation : **AMU 1986, 87**
A. Factor-V B. Factor-VIII
C. Factor-IX D. Factor-X

155. Hb is a good buffer because of : **Kerala 1994**
A. Histidine residues B. Protein nature
C. Acidic nature D. Fe molecule

156. Thrombosthenin is present in : **PGI 1988, 98**
A. Plasma B. Platelets
C. Neutrophils D. RBC's

157. Haematocrit is ratio of : **AMC 1983, 87, 99**
A. WBC to plasma B. Platelets to plasma
C. RBC's to plasma D. Total blood cells to plasma

158. Hemotocrit of venous blood is : **DNB 1989, 99**
A. 3% greater than arterial blood
B. 3 times greater than arterial blood
C. 3% less than arterial blood
D. 3 times less than arterial blood

159. H^+ is more bound to : **AMU 1985, 98**
A. Deoxygenated hemoglobin
B. Oxygenated hemoglobin
C. Both a+b equally
D. Not related to oxygenation

160. Myoglobin binds with : **AP 1985, 95**
A. 1 mol of oxygen per mol
B. 2 mol of oxygen per mol
C. 3 mol of oxygen per mol
D. 4 mol of oxygen per mol

161. Alkali resistant Hb is : **Kerala 1994, 96**
A. HbA B. HbA_2
C. HbF D. HbS

162. In anemia, the concentration of 2,3 DPG is : **DNB 1988, 98**
A. Decreased B. Increased
C. a or b D. Not changed

Ans. **153. B** **154. C** **155. A** **156. B** **157. C** **158. A**
159. A **160. A** **161. C** **162. B**

163. The commonest site of haemopoiesis in foetus is : **Delhi 1989, 90**

A. Liver B. Spleen
C. Bone marrow D. Gut

164. The number of O_2 molecules carried by on Hb molecule: **AMU 1989, 94**

A. 1 B. 2
C. 4 D. 8

165. A patient has a plasma concentration of HCO_3 of 13 m M/L and a plasma PCO_2 of 50 mm Hg. He has : **AP 1990, 99**

A. Compensated metabolic acidosis
B. Compensated respiratory acidosis
C. Respiratory acidosis and metabolic acidosis
D. Respiratory alkalosis and metabolic acidosis
E. Compensated respiratory alkalosis

166. Which one of the following statements concerning the monocyte is incorrect ? **Kerala 1989, 99**

A. More common in blood than eosinophil and basophil
B. Produced in the adult by the bone marrow and lymph nodes
C. Unlike neutrophil is rich in lipase
D. Unlike neutrophil does not accumulate outside circulation in area of inflammation

167. Which of the following statements about lymphocytes is incorrect? **Kerala 1989, 94**

A. Produced by thymus, red bone marrow, spleen and lymph nodes
B. Concentration falls in the blood abruptly and immune reaction is disturbed after removal of thymus in adult
C. Probably change into plasma cells
D. Constitute 20-40% of leukocytes

168. The normal A/G ratio in blood is : **AP 1989, 96**

A. 5 : 1 B. 2 : 1
C. 1 : 2 D. 1 : 1

169. The life span of the average erythrocyte in a new born is : **DNB 1992, 99**

A. 100 days B. 120 days
C. 160 days D. 8 months

Ans. **163. A** **164. C** **165. C** **166. D** **167. B** **168. B** **169. A**

170. The absence of anti-A and anti-Rh agglutinins in plasma means the subject is : AMU 1988,98

A. A-positive or AB-positive
B. A-negative or AB-negative
C. A-positive, AB-positive
D. Type O

171. Which one of the following represents the most potentially dangerous situation ? PGI 1988

A. Rh positive mother with 2nd Rh-negative child
B. Rh negative mother with 2nd Rh-positive child
C. Rh positive mother with 1st Rh-negative child
D. Rh negative mother with 1st Rh-positive child

172. What does characterise function of platelets ? Orissa 1991, 95

A. Form thrombus and release serotonin
B. Initiate and accelerate clot formation
C. Contribute, possibly to integrity of capillary membrane
D. All of the above

173. Increased activity of delta-amino levullinic synthetase results in: AMU 1986, 99

A. Thalasaemia B. Sickle cell anaemia
C. Porphyria D. Megaloblastic anaemia

174. In an adult man, there is about ——— hemoglobin in circulating blood : DNB 1993, 95

A. 350g B. 500g
C. 900g D. 1000g

175. Half-life of transfused platelets is : AIIMS 1987, 97

A. 4 hours B. 12 hours
C. 4 days D. 17 days

176. Cyanosis is seen if the concentration of methaemoglobin is more than __________ gm%: AIIMS 1987; AI 1998

A. 1.5 B. 2.0
C. 3.0 D. 4.0

177. Erythropoietin is increased in : Delhi 1983, 85

A. Blood loss B. High altitude
C. Exercise D. All of the above

Ans. **170. C** **171. B** **172. D** **173. C** **174. C** **175. C**
176. A **177. D**

178. The need for Vitamin B_{12} and folic acid in the formation of red blood cells is related primarily of their effects on : **AIIMS 1984, 94, 95**

A. Synthesis and release of erythropoietin from the kidney
B. Absorption of iron from the gut
C. DNA synthesis in Bone marrow
D. Hemoglobin formation in the red blood cell

179. HbE is formed due to replacement of glutamic acid at 26th position by ———— : **WB 1998, 99**

A. Glycine B. Lysine
C. Arginine D. Valine

180. Which is wrong regarding factor-VIII vWF : **WB 1998, 99**

A. Factor-VIII is produced by liver
B. vWF is produced by endothelial cell
C. vWF prevents platelet adhesion with collagen
D. Factor-VIII activates factor-X

181. Which one of the following statements regarding oxygenation and deoxygenation of haemoglobin (Hb) is correct ? **CSE 1997, 98**

A. Oxygenated Hb is a stronger acid when compared to deoxygenated Hb
B. Deoxygenated Hb is a stronger acid when compared to oxygenated Hb
C. The acidic characters of the oxygenated Hb and deoxygenated Hb are of the same magnitude
D. Since Hb is present inside the erythrocytes, its oxygenation or deoxygenation does not alter the acidic or basic character

182. Respiratory alkalosis may be produced by: **CSE 1997, 98**

A. Chronic obstructive pulmonary disease
B. Drugs causing respiratory depression
C. Hyperpnea
D. Excessive renal bicarbonate absorption

183. Factor used in the extrinsic pathway of blood coagulation is : **Delhi 1985, 98**

A. V B. VIII
C. Tissue factor-III D. X

184. In polycythemia, the increase in blood pressure is due to increase in : **PGI 1983, 95**

A. Blood volume B. Peripheral resistance
C. Thyroxin D. Renin

Ans. 178. C 179. D 180. C 181. B 182. C 183. C 184. B

185. Vitamin-K is required for the synthesis of factors : PGI 1982

A. VII B. IX
C. X D. All of the above

186. Carbonic anhydrase in RBC forms : AIIMS 1984; Delhi 1988

A. Oxy hemoglobin
B. Carboxy hemoglobin
C. HCO_3^- in blood
D. Carbamino hemoglobin

187. When osmotic fragility is normal, RBC's begin to hemolyse when suspended in saline : DNB 1989, 99

A. 0.33% B. 0.48%
C. 0.9% D. 1.2%

188. Thromboxane A2 is released mainly by the :
AIIMS 1982; AI 1990

A. Platelets B. Vascular endothelium
C. Liver D. Muscles

189. The best screening test for hemophilia is : Bihar 1991, 98

A. BT B. PT
C. PTT D. CT

190. The greatest amount of CO_2 is transported in the blood as :
Bihar 1991, 98

A. RBC's B. HCO_3
C. Carbamino-Hb D. H_2CO_3
E. Platelets

191. Blood group antigens are : PGI 1987; AI 1988, 98

A. Carried by sex chromosomes
B. Attached to plasma proteins
C. Attached to Hemoglobin molecule
D. Found in saliva

192. A reliable screening test for platelet function is :
Bihar 1991, 94, 99

A. CT B. PT
C. Thrombin time D. Clot retraction time

193. In which of the following, bleeding time is characteristically increased : AIIMS 1988, 92

A. Von Willebrand's disease
B. Hemophilia A
C. Hereditary hemolytic telangiectasia
D. Henoch-Scholein purpura

Ans. **185. D** **186. C** **187. B** **188. A** **189. C** **190. B**
191. D **192. D** **193. A**

194. Freezing point of normal human plasma is : PGI 1984, 96

A. 4°C B. 0°C

C. -0.54°C D. -1.54°C

195. For cyanosis to be manifested, the amount of reduced hemoglobin in blood, should be : AIIMS 1982; 84; AMC 1987

A. 1 gm% B. 3 gm%

C. 5 gm% D. 7 gm%

196. Iron is stored in : PGI 1984; AMC 1986; AI 1990

A. RBC

B. Reticulo endothelial system

C. Plasma

D. All of the above

197. Adult hemoglobin has chains : Delhi 1983, 88, 99

A. 2 α, 2 γ B. 2 α, 2β

C. 4α D. 2 α

198. Endothelial cells synthesize : Delhi 1987, 93, 98

A. Fibrinogen B. Factor-VIII

C. Factor-X D. Factor-XII

199. Life of R.B.C. is : Delhi 1992

A. 30 days B. 90 days

C. 120 days D. 160 days

200. The best method for estimation of Hb concentration in blood is : Delhi 1992, 99

A. Acid heamatin method

B. Alkali haematin method

C. Cyanmethhaemoglobin method

D. Any of the above

201. In vitro coagulation is initiated by factor : Delhi 1986, 92, 99

A. XII B. XI

C. X D. VII

202. Arneth Count is counting of : AIIMS 1988, 99

A. Lymphocytes

B. Lobes in neutrophilis

C. Granules in eosinophiils

D. WBC in bone marrow

203. The number of Fe atoms in one Hb molecule is : DNB 1992, 94

A. 1 B. 2

C. 4 D. 8

Ans. 194. C 195. C 196. B 197. B 198. B 199. C
200. C 201. A 202. B 203. C

204. Vitamin-B12 is essential for what aspect of blood cell reproduction : PGI 1982, 94

A. Formation of hemoglobin
B. Extrusion of the nucleus from the normoblasts
C. Formation of DNA
D. Activation of erythropoietin

205. In a person with type O blood, what type or types of agglutinins does he has in plasma : AMC 1984; UPSC 1983, 84

A. None B. Alpha
C. Beta D. Alpha and beta

206. Reticulocytes are stained with : AIIMS 1988, 99

A. Methyl violet B. Brilliant Cresyl blue
C. Sudan black D. Indigo carmine

207. Cells with more than ——— MCV/(fl) are called macrocytes : AIIMS 1983 ,94

A. 80 B. 87
C. 90 D. 95

208. Mean corpuscular diameter (nm) is : PGI 1984, 95

A. 4.1 B. 6.3
C. 7.2 D. 7.5

209. What is the maximum concentration of hemoglobin normally found in red blood cells : PGI 1986, 96

A. 5 per cent B. 10 per cent
C. 16 per cent D. 20 per cent
E. 34 per cent

210. When infection occurs a tissue, what type of white blood cells is first attracted from the blood into the tissue by the process of chemotaxis : PGI 1980, 98

A. Neutrophilis B. Monocytes
C. Eosinophilis D. Basophils

211. What is the first important event in hemostasis following severe tissue injury : AIIMS 1986, 95

A. Blood coagulation
B. Formation of a platelet plug
C. Vascular spasm
D. Formation of thromboplastin

212. The conversion of fibrinogen into fibrin occurs by : Delhi 1987, 89, 99

A. Prothrombin B. Thrombin
C. Thrombophlebitis D. Platelets

Ans. **204. C** **205. D** **206. B** **207. D** **208. D** **209. E**
210. A **211. C** **212. B**

213. Esoinophilia is caused by following except : **AIIMS 1993, 94**
A. Stress B. Aspirin
C. PAN D. Ascariasis

214. Platelets growth factor are synthesized by : **Delhi 1993, 95**
A. Glial cells B. Endothelium
C. Fibroblasts D. All of the above

215. The theory of blood flow and lymph drainage is by: **PGI 1995, 96**
A. Starling B. Avagadro
C. Mitchell D. Bergili via vitalis

216. Complete erythropoisis occurs in ——— days : **DNB 1994, 96**
A. 3 B. 7
C. 14 D. 20

217. In a 30 years old man function of which bone marrow is not important for blood formation : **Rajasthan 1994, 99**
A. Vertebral B. Ribs
C. Sternum D. Shaft of humerus

218. Fetal RBC's differ from Adult RBC's by following except : **AIIMS 1997, 99**
A. Fetal RBC's bigger
B. More 2-3 DPG in foetal RBC's
C. Foetal RBC's have shorter life span
D. Less of carbonic anhydrase

219. The affinity of oxygen for Hb increased with fall in pH. This is called : **Orissa 1999**
A. Bain bridge effect B. Bohr's effect
C. Haldane effect D. Herring effect

220. ↑ blood vicosity & slow circulation causes : **TN 1999**
A. RBC Rouleux formation
B. ↑ Plasma skimming
C. ↑ number of RBC is capillaries
D. ↑ WBC's count

221. Glycophorin is seen in : **PGI 1999**
A. Enterocyte B. Erythrocyte
C. Lymphocyte D. Hepatocyte

222. Clotting factor which is not formed by liver : **PGI 1999**
A. 10 B. 7
C. 8 D. 2

Ans. **213. A** **214. D** **215. A** **216. B** **217. D** **218. B**
219. B **220. A** **221. B** **222. C**

223. A haematocrit of 41% in the sample of blood analyzed means : **TNPSC 1996**

A. 41% of the blood volume is the plasma
B. 41% of the total blood volume is made up of plasma
C. 41% of the blood volume is the red blood cells
D. 41% of the toal blood volume is made up of red and white blood cells and platelets

224. Increased osmotic fragility is found in the following except : **UP 1999**

A. Spectrin deficiency
B. G-6 PD deficiency
C. Hereditary hemolytic anemia
D. Sickle cell disease

225. When a blood vessel wall is injured, all of the following promote platelet activation except : **Kerala 2000**

A. Prostacyclin
B. Collagen
C. ADP
D. Thrombin
E. von Willebrand factor

226. Erythropoietin is secreted by following except : **PGI 2000**

A. Hemangioblastoma
B. Hepatoma
C. Renal cell carcinoma
D. Adrenocortical tumours

227. Blood is non-Newtonian fluid because : **AI 2001**

A. Viscosity changes with velosity
B. Density changes with velocity
C. Density does not change with velocity
D. Viscosity does not change with velocity

228. Cyanosis is caused by : **Rohtak 2001**

A. Reduced Hb above 7.5 gm/dl
B. Met. Hb above 1.5 g/dl
C. Sulph. Hb above 0.5
D. All of the above

229. Shape of RBC is maintained by : **AIIMS 2002**

A. Integrin
B. Spectrin
C. Globin
D. Ankyrin

Ans. 223. C 224. D 225. A 226. D 227. A 228. D 229. B

230. A shift of posture from supine to upright posture is associated with cardiovascular adjustments. Which of the following is not true in this context : AIIMS 2003

A. Rise in central venous pressure.
B. Rise in heart rate.
C. Decrease in cardiac output.
D. Decrease in stroke volume.

231. Following are correct about potassium balance except : AIIMS 2003

A. Most of potassium is intracellular
B. Three quarter of the total body potassium is found in skeletal muscle.
C. Intracellular potassium is released into extra-cellular space in response to severe injury or surgical stress.
D. Acidosis leads to movement of potassium from extracellular to intracellular fluid compartment.

232. Which of the following is procoagulation protein? AI 2004

A. Thrombomodulin B. Protein-C
C. Protein-S D. Thrombin

233. All endothelial cells produce thrombomodulin except those found in : AI 2005

A. Hepatic circulation
B. Cutaneous circulation
C. Cerebral microcirculation
D. Renal circulation

234. The type of hemoglobin that has least affinity for 2,3 - Diphospho-glycerate (2,3-DPG) or (2,3-BPG) is : AI 2005

A. HbA B. HbF
C. HbB D. HbA_2

235. Heme is converted to bilirubin mainly in : AI 2005

A. Kidney B. Liver
C. Spleen D. Bone marrow

236. Hb is measured by following methods except : AIIMS 2007

A. Drabkin's
B. Sahli's
C. Spectrophotometery
D. Wintrobe's

237. The substance that is present in both serum and plasma is : AI 2007

A. Fibrinogen B. Factor - VII
C. Factor-V D. Factor-II

Ans. 230. A 231. D 232. D 233. C 234. B 235. C
236. D 237. B

238. Site of RBC formation in 20 years old healthy male is : **AI 2007**

A. Flat bones B. Long bones
C. Liver D. Yolk sac

239. Which of the following helps in bridging the fibrin in a clot and stabilizing the clot? **AI 2008**

A. Factor-III B. Factor-V
C. Factor-VIII D. Factor-XIII

Ans. 238. A 239. D

EXPLANATIONS OF PHYSIOLOGICAL ASPECTS

1. Ans. — C Decreased oncotic pressure in capillaries

* **The rate of filtration at any point along a capillary depends on a balance of forces sometimes called the Starling forces after the physiologist who first described their operation in detail.**

* **One of these forces is the hydrostatic pressure gradient (the hydrostatic pressure in the capillary minus the hydrostatic pressure of the interstitial fluid) at the point. The interstitial fluid pressure varies from one organ to another, and there is considerable evidence that it is subatmospheric (about - 2 mmIIg) in subcutaneous tissue. It is positive in the liver and kidneys and is as high as 6 mm Hg in the brain.**

* **The other force is the osmotic pressure gradient across the capillary wall (colloid osmotic pressure of plasma minus colloid osmotic pressure of interstitial fluid). This component is directed inward. Thus :**

  k = capillary filtration coefficient

  pc= capillary hydrostatic pressure

  p1 = interstitial hydrostatic pressure

  ***c = capillary colloid osmotic pressure**

  Pie1 = interstitial colloid osmotic pressure

  pi is usually negligible, so the osmotic pressure gradient (pc-p1) usually equals the oncotic pressure.

* **The capillary filtration coefficient takes into account, and is proportionate to the permeability of the capillary wall and the area available for filtration.**

* **Fluid moves into the interstitial space at the arteriolar end of the capillary, where the filtration pressure across its wall exceeds the oncotic pressure, and into the capillary at the venular end, where the oncotic pressure exceeds the filtration pressure.**
* **In other capillaries, the balance of Starling force is different and, for example, fluid moves out of almost the entire length of the capillaries in the renal glomeruli. On the other hand, fluid moves into the capillaries through almost their entire length in the intestines.**

2. Ans.— D 420.4 mm Hg

The data provided in the question is :

* **PaO_2 —> 100 mm Hg**
* **$PaCO_2$ —> 40 mm Hg**
* **FiO_2 —> 8 mm Hg**

What is FIO_2?

FIO is the fraction of oxygen in inspired air.

At sea level (760 mm Hg pressure), the composition of the air is roughly

O_2 —>20%

N_2 —>80%

So FiO_2 is $\frac{20}{100} = .2$

In the question, the child is being ventilated with 80% Oxygen

So the FiO_2 will be $= \frac{80}{100} .8$

Now, PAO_2 can be calculated by Alveolar gas equation

$$PAO_2 = FIO_2 \times (Ps - PH_2O) - \frac{PaCO_2}{R}$$

Where

* **PAO2 —> PO2 of the alveolar air**
* **FIO2 —> Fraction of O2 in the air**
* **PB—> Barometric pressure (N is 760 mm Hg)**
* **PH2O—> Water vapour pressure (N is 47 mm H_2O)**
* **PaCO2 —> 40**

Substituting these values

$PAO_2 = .8 \times (760\text{-}47) - 40/.8$

= 520.4 mm Hg

* **Therefore $PAO_2 - PaO_2$ = (520.4 mmg Hg - 100 mm Hg) = 420.4 mm Hg**

3. Ans. — C Multiple Myeloma

In Multiple myeloma M proteins increase in the blood, this may cause cryoglobulinemia which leads to increase in viscosity of the blood.

Viscosity of the blood depends upon:

a) Hematocrit

b) Composition of the plasma

a) Hematocrit - (percentage of the volume of the blood occupied by red blood cells).

*** Increase in hematocrit**

(e.g. Polycythemia)—>Increase in viscosity

*** Decrease in hematocrit**

(e.g.) Anemia —> Decrease in viscosity

b) Composition of the plasma - Composition of the plasma depends upon the presence of plasma proteins such as immunoglobulins and the resistance of the cells to deformation.

*** Increase in plasma protein**

(immunoglobulin) —> Increase in viscosity e.g. multiple myeloma.

*** Increase in resistance of cells to:**

deformation —> Increase in viscosity e.g. hereditary spherocytosis.

4. Ans. — A Large veins

*** The velocity of blood is inversely proportional to the total cross-sectional area at that point.**

*** Thus, the velocity of blood is high in aorta, declines steadily in the smaller arteries and is lowest in the capillaries. (The capillaries have 1000 times the total cross-sectional area of the aorta) The velocity of blood flow increases again as the blood enter the veins and is relatively high again in the vena cava, although not so high as in the aorta.**

5. Ans. — C Cyanide poisoning

*** This type of hypoxia where the oxygen content of blood is normal, but the tissue is unable to utilizes the oxygen due to failure of its cellular metabolic processes is known as histotoxic hypoxia.**

- **The best known cause of histotoxic hypoxia is cyanide poisoning, which inhibits cytochrome oxidase.**
- **Another example of histotoxic hypoxia is beri-beri, where several important steps in tissue utilization of oxygen are compromised because of vitamin-B Deficiency.**

Other Types of Hypoxia :

a. Hypoxic hypoxia.

— When there is poor availability of O_2 for diffussion to the pulmonary capillaries.

— There is inadequate PO_2 in arterial blood.

b. Anemic hypoxia

— When the hypoxia is due to quantitative or qualitative deficiency of Hb.

— The oxygen content of arterial blood is almost all bound to Hb. In the presence of severe anemia or CO poisoning, the oxygen content of blood will fall, even though the PO2 of arterial blood will remain normal.

c. Stagnant or circulatory hypoxia.

— When the hypoxia is due to poor velocity of blood.

— In cases of circulatory failure even though the oxygen content of arterial blood may be adequate, delivery to the tissue is not.

6. Ans.— D. Venules
7. Ans.— C. Capillaries
8. Ans.— E. Veins
9. Ans.— C. Capillaries
10. Ans.— C. Capillaries
11. Ans.— C. 2000

The rate of flow ($F=P_1-P_2$) depends upon the resistance

$$Fa\frac{1}{R}$$

12. Ans.— C. Air embolism
13. Ans.— A. Histotoxic hypoxia
14. Ans.— A. Carboxy hemoglobin
15. Ans.— C. 210
16. Ans.— A. Hypoxic
17. Ans.— D. Carbon monoxide poisoning
18. Ans.— A. Have blood flow rate similar to that of brain

19. Ans.— D. They can manufacture immunoglobulins
20. Ans.— A. Shifting affinity for oxygen
21. Ans.— D. O2 content of blood from right ventricle
22. Ans.— A. In pulmonary capillaries
23. Ans.— D. Have a discontinuous basement membrane
24. Ans.— B. Are not found in skeletal muscle
25. Ans.— C. Did not enter cells of body
26. Ans.— A. Sample from peripheral artery
Pulse pressure is the difference between the systolic and diastolic pressures, is normally about 50 mmHg.
27. Ans.— D. Stagnant anoxia
28. Ans.— C. Histotoxic anoxia
29. Ans.— D. Stagnant anoxia
30. Ans.— B. Anoxic anoxia
31. Ans.— B. Anoxic anoxia
32. Ans.— A. Anaemic anoxia
33. Ans.— A. Anaemic anoxia
34. Ans.— D. Peripheral vascular resistance
35. Ans.— C. Vasodilator metabolites
Lactate is important
36. Ans.— C. Law of Laplace
Law of Laplace states that tension in the wall of a cylinder (T) is equal to the product of the transmural pressure (P) and the radius (r) divided by wall thickness (w) i.e. ($T = Pr/w$).
37. Ans.— B. Systemic artery
38. Ans.— D. R_4
39. Ans.— C. Decreased haematocrit
40. Ans.— C. Raised systolic blood pressure
41. Ans.— D. Lying down
42. Ans.— B. Muscle
43. Ans.— C. Greater than the pulse pressure in the upper aorta
44. Ans.— C. HCO_3^-
45. Ans.— B. 1, 3, 2, 4
46. Ans.— C. 0.2
47. Ans.— A. Osmal
48. Ans.— A. Capillaries
49. Ans.— C. ↓ Lactate
A fall in temperature or a rise in pH also shifts the curve to left. Fall in 2, 3 DPG concentration also shifts the curve to left.

50. Ans.— B. Hyperthermia
It is forms carboxyhemoglobin
51. Ans.— C. Extrusion of Na
52. Ans.— B. Pottassium
53. Ans.— A. Raised 2-3 DPG
A rise of temperature or a fall in pH also shifts the oxygen dissociation curve to right.
54. Ans.— D. Tachynoea
55. Ans.— B. 25-50 mm Hg
56. Ans.— D. All of the above
57. Ans.— B. 97%
58. Ans.— C. 40 46 75
59. Ans.— C. 70 fold
60. Ans.— C. 5 % of cardiac output
Heart muscle has mass of 0.3 Kg and blood flow of 250 mL/min or 84 mL/100g/min. It receives 4.7% of cardiac output and 11.6% of total oxygen consumption.
61. Ans.— A. Unknown
62. Ans.— C. 5 mmHg in man
63. Ans.— A. 500 ml/min
64. Ans.— A. 2 : 1
65. Ans.— D. Increased cardiac activity
66. Ans.— D. Arterioles
67. Ans.— B. Skeletal muscle
68. Ans.— C. Heart muscle
69. Ans.— B. Skeletal muscle
70. Ans.— C. Heart
71. Ans.— B. 0.07
72. Ans.— A. Liver
Weight of liver is 1.2 -1.5 kg
73. Ans.— A. Kidneys
74. Ans.— C. Atrial fibrillation
75. Ans.— C. 25-28 mm/L
76. Ans.— C. 15 sec
77. Ans.— C. 4.3 ml
78. Ans.— A. Circulating angiotensin-II
79. Ans.— A. Dilate
Axon reflex is a response in which impulse initiated in sensory nerves by the injury are relayed antidromically down other branches of the sensory nerve fibres.
80. Ans.— D. pH of blood

81. Ans.— C. Increased renal arterial blood flow
82. Ans.— D. Increased venous pressure
83. Ans.— E. A and C
84. Ans.— NONE
85. Ans.— D. Capillaries
86. Ans.— C. It is mainly produced by the bone marrow
87. Ans.— D. 30 mm Hg
88. Ans.— D. Heart rate increases
89. Ans.— C. Emotional shock
90. Ans.— D. Axon reflex
91. Ans.— D. Isovolumetric contraction

At the start of ventricular systole, the mitral and tricuspid valves close, ventricular muscle initially shortens relatively little but intraventricular pressure rises sharply as the myocardium presses on the blood in the ventricle. This period of isovolumetric (isovolumic, isometric) ventricular contraction lasts about 0.05 sec. until the pressures in the left and right ventricles exceed the pressures in the aortic and pulmonary valves open.

92. Ans.— B. Shift of intracellular fluid to extracellular space
93. Ans.— D. 1 alone is correct
94. Ans.— D. Brain, heart, kidney
95. Ans.— D. All of the above
96. Ans.— A. Blood velocity in capillary is greater than large vein
97. Ans.— D. Histotoxic hypoxia
98. Ans.— A. ↓ Cellular respiration
99. Ans.— C. Kidneys
100. Ans.— B. Resistance low, capillary pressure low
101 Ans.— C. Coronary circulation

Coronary circulation is not affected in exercise in a normal person

102. Ans.— D. Hyperthermia
103. Ans.— B. 500-600 ml
104. Ans.— B. Large ↑ Pulm. Artery pressure
105. Ans.— B. 20-30
106. Ans.— D. Cerebral blood flow will not change appreciably
107. Ans.— B. Increased tone of capacitance veins

108. Ans.— B. increased tone of capacitance veins

109. Ans.— C. Cerebrum.
Autoregulation of blood flow is typically seen in brain

110. Ans.— B. V/Q ratio
According to Fick principle, the blood flow of any organ can be measured by determining the amount of a given substance (Qx) removed from the blood stream by the organ per unit of time and dividing that value by the difference between the concentration of the substance in arterial blow and concentration in venous blood from organ.

111. Ans.— A. Liver>Kidney>brain>heart

112. Ans.— A. Reflex bradycardia

113. Ans.— A. 1, 2 and 3

114. Ans.— A. Nitric oxide

115. Ans.— C. Intestine

116. Ans.— A. Synthesized from arginine

117. Ans.— B. Slight increase in HR, normal BP

118. Ans.— D. Low mol. wt. high concentration

119. Ans.— C. Increased rate of blood flow

120. Ans.— C. 5 mm/sec
Velocity of blood is v = Q/A

121. Ans.— A. Anaemic hypoxia

122. Ans.— B. Redistribution of body fluids

123. Ans.— A. Hypertension

124. Ans.— A. 53

125. Ans.— B. Positive feedback stabilizes system

126. Ans.— A. Proteoglycans

127. Ans.— D. Carotid body
The blood flow in each 2 mg of carotid body about 0.04 mL/min or 2000 mL/100 gm of tissue/min compared to 100 g/min of 54 ml in brain and 420 mL in the kidneys.

128. Ans.— B. Small arteries

129. Ans.— D. 100 mm Hg

$$\text{Pressure} = \frac{\text{Concentration of dissolved gas}}{\text{Solubility coefficients}}$$

When pressure is expressed in atmospheric (1 atmospheric = 760 mmHg) and conc is expressed in volume of gas dissolved in each volume of water, the solubility coefficient for gases at body temperature.

Gases	Solubility coefficient
O_2	0.025
CO_2	0.57
CO	0.018
N_2	0.012
He	0.008

In this question –

Conc. of O_2 in blood = 0.0025 ml/ml

= 2.5 ml/L

$$O_2 \text{ tension} = \frac{\text{Conc. of } O_2}{\text{Solubility coefficient}}$$

$$= \frac{2.5}{0.025}$$

= 100 mmHg

130. Ans.— D. Vascular endothelium is smooth and coated with glycocalyx

- Intact endothelial cells serves primarily to inhibit platelet adherence and blood clotting.
- Injury or activation of endothelial cells, however, results in a procoagulant phenotype that augments local clot formation.

Role of vascular endothelium in hemostasis

- The vascular endothelium acts as a barrier between the thrombogenic subendothelial tissue and the blood.
- The smoothness of endothelial cells hinder platelet aggregation.
- They manufactures heparan and a_2 macroglobulin which are coagulation inhibitors.
- These cells manufactures PHI_2 (prostacyclin) which opposes platelet aggregation.

Factors opposing coagulation, existing clots and platelets plugging and occurring naturally

A. Opposing coagulation
- **Antithrombin-III**
- **Heparin**
- **Heparan**
- **a_2 macroglobulin**
- **Protein-C**

B. Causing lysis of existing clot
- **Plasminogen activators**

C. Opposing platelet aggregation
- **Endoperoxidase from platelets**
- **Prostacyclin**

Note

- **Vit-K dependent factor 2, 7, 9, 10, CS**
- **Factor-II (prothrombin), VII, IX, and X**
- **Protein-C and Protein-S**
- **Factors synthesis by liver 2, 7, 9, 10, CS + 1, 5, 11**
- **Factor-I (fibrinogen), II (Prothrombin), V, VII, IX, X, XI**
- **Protein-C and protein-S**
- **Antithrombin-III and heparin**

131. Ans.— D. Hypoventilation

DISORDER WHICH LOWERS ARTERIAL PO2

1. **Hypoventilation**
2. **Diffusion defects**
3. **Low ventilation perfusion ratio**
4. **Arteriovenous shunts**
5. **Pump failure (ventilatory failure)**
   - **Fatigue**
   - **Mechanical defects**
   - **Depression of respiratory controller in Brain**

* **Anemic hypoxia : Arterial PO2 is normal**

* **CO poisoning : PO2 remains normal**

* **Moderate excercise : Almost normal PO2 (Due to increase in pulmonary ventilation, perfusion and diffusion)**

132. Ans.— B. Brain

"Exposure to high concentration of CO2 is associated with marked cutaneous and cerebral vasodilatation but there is vasoconstriction elsewhere and usually a slow rise in blood pressure".

133. Ans.— B. Arterioles

"Arterioles, metarterioles and precapillary sphincters are rich in smooth muscle, contraction of which is subject of REGULATORY MECHANISM."

* The smooth muscle of these segments respond to stretch, temperature and other neurohumoral and chemical factors. (given in the previous ques.)
* Response to these factors help in matching blood flow to organs with their requirement.

134. Ans.— D. Bicarbonate

"Transport in the form of Bicarbonate accounts for 70% of carbon dioxide transport."

CO_2 in each deciletre of Blood

1. In HCO_3 (Bicarbonate)	43. 8 mL
2. In Carbamino compounds	2.6 mL
3. Dissolved in Blood	2.6 mL

Total CO_2

135. Ans.— D. 30 mmHg

136. Ans.— A. ↓ Capillary permeability

The flow rate in adult is

Pressure gradient	Diameter of vessel	Flow rate
P= 100 mm Hg	1 mm	1ml/min
P= 100 mm Hg	2 mm	16 ml/min
P=100 mm Hg	4 mm	256 ml/min

This is determined by Poiseuille's law

137. Ans.— A. Plasma

$$\text{Volume} \times \frac{100}{100-0.87\ \text{haematocrit}}$$

138. Ans.— D. Muscle

139. Ans.— C. 5-6 times more that of water

Velocity (V) is proportionate to flow (Q) divided by the area of conduit (A) i.e. V=Q/A. Therefore Q=AV, and if flow stays constant, in A.

140. Ans.— B. **Venous return to the heart rises immediately**

On changing position from standing to lying, there is an increase in venous return to the heart and an increase in the B.P. in the carotid sinus and aortic arch. This leads to decrease in heart rate. There is an increase in arterial pressure at head level but because of prominent autoregulation in the brain blood flow remains relatively normal. In the lying down position blood flow to the apices increase.

141. Ans.— B. **Type of fluid administered**

O_2 delivery to a particular tissue depends on :

* **amount of O_2 entering the lungs**
* **the adequacy of pulmonary gas exchange**
* **the blood flow to the tissues**
* - **cardiac output**
  - **degree of constriction of the vascular bed in the tissue**
* **the capacity of blood of carry O_2**
  - **the amount of dissolved O_2 in plasma**
  - **the amount of hemoglobin**
  - **the affinity of the hemoglobin for O_2**

142. Ans.— B. **Increased by massaging the foot**

As evident, when an individual rises from the supine to standing position the lymphatic flow from the foot will decrease and not increase, due to gravity.

If we massage the foot we will force the lymphatic flow (as well as venous return), by forcing the lymph to enter the lymphatic vessels.

143. Ans.— B. **Presence of deep facial planes (most probably)**

* **So, the factors which keeps blood flowing in the veins towards the heart are :**

1. **Pumping action of the heart (arterial blood pressure)**
2. **Heartbeat (also contributes to the arterial blood pressure)**
3. **The increase in the negative intrathoracic pressure during each inspiration**
4. **Contractions of skeletal muscles that compress the veins (muscle pump).**

144. Ans.— C. X

145. Ans.— C. 34

MCHC (g/dL) is Hb x 100. It is 34 in both male and females.

MCH is Hb x 10 ———— (It is 29) and MCV is :

Hematocrit
——————
RBC count

Hct x 100
——————— (10^6 mL) (It is 87)
RBC count

146. Ans.— C. Trauma

147. Ans.— B. EDTA

148. Ans.— D. All of the above

149. Ans.— B. Intermediate normoblast

150. Ans.— D. None of the above

151. Ans.— B. 9-12 days

Lifespan of transfused platelets is only 4 days.

152. Ans.— B. K^+ than Na^+

153. Ans.— B. Contractile protein

154. Ans.— C. Factor-IX

155. Ans.— A. Histidine residues

156. Ans.— B. Platelets

157. Ans.— C. RBC's to plasma See Ques. 2

158. Ans.— A. 3% greater than arterial blood

159. Ans.— A. Deoxygenated hemoglobin

160. Ans.— A. 1 mol of oxygen per mol

161. Ans.— C. HbF

162. Ans.— B. Increased

The concentration of 2,3 diphos-phoglycerate (DPG or 2,3 DPG) is plentiful in red cells. It is formed from 3-phospho-glyceraldehyde, which is a product of glycolysis via Embden-Meyerhof pathway. One mole of deoxyhemoglobin binds 1 mol of 2,3 DPG. pH also affects concentration of 2,3 OPG in red cells. Acidosis inhibits red cell glycolysis and thus fall in 2,3 DPG whereas thyroid hormones, GH and androgens increase concentration of 2,3 DPG. High altitude also increases concentration of 2,3 DPG. Anemia and chronic hypoxia also increase 2,3 DPG.

163. Ans.— A. Liver

164. Ans.— C. 4

165. Ans.— C. Respiratory acidosis and metabolic acidosis

166. Ans.— D. Unlike neutrophil does not accumulate outside circulation in area of inflammation

167. Ans.— B. Constration falls in the blood abruptly and immune reaction is disturbed after removal of thymus in adult.

168. Ans.— B. 2 : 1
It is reversed in malnutrition

169. Ans.— A. 100 days
Lifespan of RBC's in adult is 120 days whereas that in tranfused blood is 90 days.

170. Ans.— C. A-positive, AB-positive

171. Ans.— B. Rh negative mother with 2nd Rh-positive child

172. Ans.— D. All of the above

173. Ans.— C. Porphyria
It is used in acute intermittent porphyria

174. Ans.— C. 900g

175. Ans.— C. 4 days

176. Ans.— A. 1.5
Reduced hemoglobin concentration of blood in capillaries is more than 5 gm/dL also causes cyanosis.

177. Ans.— D. All of the above

178. Ans.— C. DNA synthesis in Bone marrow

179. Ans.— D. Valine

180. Ans.— C. vWF prevents platelet adhesion with collagen

181. Ans.— B. Deoxygenated Hb is a stronger acid when compared to oxygenated Hb

182. Ans.— C. Hyperpnea

183. Ans.— C. Tissue factor III

184. Ans.— B. Peripheral resistance

185. Ans.— D. All of the above

186. Ans.— C. HCO_3^- in blood
Carbonic anhydrase inhibitor is used as an antacid, antiepileptic and as a diuretic

187. Ans.— B. 0.48%

188. Ans.— A. Platelets

189. Ans.— C. PTT
PTT is best test whereas for platelet function, best is clot retraction time.

190. Ans.— B. HCO_3

191. Ans.— D. Found in saliva

192. Ans.— D. Clot retraction time
193. Ans.— A. Von Willebrand's disease
194. Ans.— C. -0.54°C
195. Ans.— C. 5 gm%
196. Ans.— B. Reticulo endothelial system
RES maximally stores Iron
197. Ans.— B. 2α, 2β
198. Ans.— B. Factor-VIII
Factors II, VII, IX and X are synthesized by Liver and serum or plasma concentration is 20 mg/dL.
199. Ans.— C. 120 days
200. Ans.— C. Cyammethhaemoglobin method
201. Ans.— A. XII
202. Ans.— B. Lobes in neutrophilis
203. Ans.— C. 4
204. Ans.— C. Formation of DNA
205. Ans.— D. Alpha and beta
206. Ans.— B. Brilliant Creasyl blue
207. Ans.— D. 95
208. Ans.— D. 7.5
Mean corpuscular or cell diameter is mean diameter of 500 cells in smear. In males and females, it is 7.5.
209. Ans.— E. 34 per cent
210. Ans.— A. Neutrophilis
211. Ans.— C. Vascular spasm
212. Ans.— B. Thrombin
213. Ans.— A. Stress
It is typically raised in filariasis and allergy.
214. Ans.— D. All of the above
215. Ans.— A. Starling
216. Ans.— B. 7
217. Ans.— D. Shaft of humerus
218. Ans.— B. More 2-3 DPG in foetal RBC's
219. Ans.— B. Bohr's effect
Bohr's effect is closely related to the fact that deoxygenated hemoglobin binds H^+ more actively than does oxyhemoglobin. The pH of blood falls as its CO2 content increases.
220. Ans.— A. RBC Rouleux formation
221. Ans.— B. Erythrocyte

222. Ans.— C. 8
223. Ans.— C. 41% of the blood volume is the red blood cells
224. Ans.— D. Sickle cell disease
225. Ans.— A. Prostacyclin
226. Ans.— D. Adrenocortical tumours
Erythropoietin is a glycoprotein that contains 165 amino acid residues and four oligosaccharide chains that are necessary for its activity a vivo. Its blood level is markedly increased in anemia.
227. Ans.— A. Viscosity changes with velosity
228. Ans.— D. All of the above
229. Ans.— B. Spectrin
The membrane skeleton is formed by part of spectrin and is anchored is transmembrane protein band 3 by the protein ankyrin.
230. Ans.— A. Rise in central venous pressure.
231. Ans.— D. Acidosis leads to movement of potassium from extra-cellular to intracellular fluid compartment.
232. Ans.— D. Thrombin
- In the circulating blood, thrombin is a procoagulant that activates factors-V and VII.
- When thrombin kinds to thrombomodulin (thrombin-binding protein), it becomes an anticoagulant in that the thrombomodulin thrombin complex activates protein-C.
- Activated protein -C, along with its cofactor protein S, inactivates factor-V and VII and inactivates an inhibitor of tissue plaminogen activator, increasing the formation of plasmin (fibrinolysin).

233. Ans.— C. Cerebral microcirculation
"All endothelial cells except those in the cerebral microcirculation produce thrombomodulin a thrombin binding protein and express it on their surface."
234. Ans.— B. HbF
"It is worth nothing that does not combine with foetal haemoglobin (HbF).
- That is perhaps one reason why HbF has greater affinity for oxygen than adult Hb (HbA)
- The difference in affinity has great physiological significance because it is responsible for the transfer of oxygen from the mother to the foetus when their circulations come in intimate contact in the placenta.

235. Ans.— C. Spleen

Bilirubin (0.2 to 0.3 gm/day) production from here

Mononuclear phagocytic system	
1. Spleen	1. Hepatic heme
Bone marrow	
2. Liver (premature destruction of cytochrome)	2. Hemoproteins (e.g. p-450 newly formed R.B.C.)

- Cells of the reticuloendothelial system degrades hemoglobin from wornout RBC. The porphyrin is converted into the yellow pigment bilirubin.
- The insoluble bilirubin is released into the blood, where it is carried to the liver tightly bound to plasma albumin.
- Spleen is the primary site for extravascular hemolysis.

236. Ans.— D. Wintrobe's

In Drabkin's method hemoglobin is converted to cyanmethaemoglobin by Drabkin's reagent (NaHCO3, potassium cyanide, potassium ferricyanide in distilled water) and the absorbance is measured in a photo electric colorimeter. In Sahli's method the amount of hemoglobin can be estimated by conversion of known volume of blood into acid-hematin by addition of dilute HCl and subsequent comparison of the color of solution with a suitable standard. Spectrophotometery or photoelectric colorimetery—most common is the Drabkin's method. Wintrobe's method is used to determine PCV (or Hct) and ESR.

237. Ans.— B Factor VI

Serum has essentially the same composition as plasma except that its fibrinogen and clotting factors-II, V and VIII have been removed and it has higher serotonin content because of the breakdown of platelets during clotting.

238. Ans.— A Flat bones

Beyond the age of 20 years most red cells continue to be produced in the marrow of membranous bones such as the vertebrae, sternum, ribs and ilia (Flat bones).

The marrow of long bones (except for proximal portions of humeri and tibia) becomes quite fatty & produces no more RBC after the age of 20 years.

Flat bones is thus the single best site of erythropoesis after the age of 20 years.

239. Ans.— D Factor-XIII

- **The fibrin is initially a loose mesh of interlacing strands.**
- **It is converted by the formation of covalent cross-linkages to a dense tight aggregate (stabilization).**
- **This latter reaction is catalyzed by activated factor-XIII and requires Ca^{2+}.**

PHARMACOLOGICAL ASPECTS

IMPORTANT TEXT FOR PHARMACOLOGICAL ASPECTS

HAEMATOLOGICAL ADVERSE DRUG MANIFESTATIONS

(I) Agranulocytosis

Aprindine
Captopril
Carbimazole
Cefataxime
Chloramphenicol
Clozapine
Co-trimoxazole
Cytotoxics
Gold salts
Indometacin
Metronidazole
Oxyphenbutazone
Phenothiazines
Phenylbutazone
Phenylthiouracil
Sulfonamides
Tolbutamide
Tricyclic Antidepressant

II) Churg-Strauss Syndrome

Flurticosane propionate
Flurticosane
Montelukast
Zafirlukast

III) Clotting or Bleeding Abnormalities

Cefamandole
Cefoperazone
Ketorolac
Mezlocillin
Moxalactum
Piperacillin
Valproic Acid

IV) Eosinophilia

Aminosalicylic acid
Chlorpropamide
Erythromycin estolate
Imipramine
L-Tryptophan
Methotrexate
Montelukast
Nitrofurantoin
Procarbazine
Sulfonamides
Zafirlukast

V) Hemolytic Anemia

Aminosalicylic acid
Cephalosporins
Chlorpromazine
Dapsone

Insulin
Isoniazid
Levodopa
Mefenamic acid
Melphalan
Methyldopa
Penicillins
Phenacetin
Procainamide
Quinidine
Rifampicin
Sulfonamides

VI) **Hemolytic Anaemia (in G-6-PD deficiency)**
Aminosalicylic acid
Antimalarials e.g. primaquine
Aspirin
Chloramphenicol
Co-trimoxazole
Dapsone
Nalidixic acid
Nitrofurantoin
Phenacetin
Probenecid
Procainamide
Quinidine
Sulfonamides
Vitamin-C
Vitamin-K

VII) **Leukocytosis**
Glucocorticoids
Lithium

VIII) **Lymphadenopathy**
Phenytoin
Primidone

IX) **Megaloblastic Anemia**
Co-trimoxazole
Folate antagonists
Nitrous oxide (repeated or prolonged exposure)
Oral contraceptives
Phenobarbital
Phenytoin
Primidone
Triamterene
Trimethophan

X) **Pancytopenia (aplastic anemia)**
Carbamazepine
Carbimazole
Chloramphenicol
Cytotoxics
Felbamate
Gold salts
Mepacrine
Mephenytoin
Oxyphenbutazone
Phenylbutazone
Phenytoin
Potassium perchlorate
Quinacrine
Sulfonamide
Thiazides
Ticlopidine
Trimethadione
Zidovadine (AZT)

XI) **Pure red cell asplasia**
Azathioprine
Chlorpropamide
Isoniazid
Phenytoin

XII) **Thrombocytopenia (see also pancytofenia)**
Acetazolamide
Aspirin
Carbamazepine
Carbenecillin

Chlorpropamide
Chlorthalidone
Co-trimoxazole
Digitoxin
Furosemide
Gold salts
Heparin
Indometacin
Isoniazid
Methyldopa
Moxalactum
Novobiocin
Oxyphenbutazone
Phenylbutazone
Phenytoin and other hydantoins
Quinidine
Quinine
Thiazides
Ticarcillin

XIII) TTP

Ticlopidine

MCQ'S FOR PHARMACOLOGICAL ASPECTS

1. **Average amount of total body iron in an adult is ______ gms :** **AIIMS 1992, 98**
   A. 2 B. 3.5
   C. 5 D. 6
2. **Which of the following preparation has the maximum iron content :** **AMC 1997**
   A. Ferrous sulphate B. Ferrous gluconate
   C. Ferrous fumarate D. Colloidal ferric hydroxide
3. **Iron dextran preparation has the following differences in comparison to iron sorbitol citric acid complex except one :** **AMU 1996**
   A. High molecular weight
   B. Can be given I/M or I/V
   C. About 20% excreted in urine
   D. Not bound to transferrin
4. **Adverse effects of parenteral iron preparations are the following except :** **DNB 1999**
   A. Joint pains B. Palpitations
   C. Constipation D. Metallic taste
5. **Iron therapy is extended for _____ months after attainment of normal Hb level :** **Delhi 1990, 94**
   A. 1-2 B. 2-4
   C. 4-6 D. 6-9
6. **Following are manifestations of acute iron poisoning except one :** **AIIMS 1995, 97, 2001**
   A. Cyanosis B. Dehydration
   C. Alkalosis D. Convulsions
7. **The dose of desferrioxamine in acute iron poisoning is ______ mg/Kg:** **PGI 1995, AIIMS 1998**
   A. 20 B. 30
   C. 50 D. 70

Ans. **1. B** **2. D** **3. C** **4. C** **5. B** **6. C** **7. C**

8. **The prophylactic dose of copper is _____ mg/d :** **UPSC 1986, AIIMS 1999**
A. 0.05 B. 0.1
C. 2.0 D. 5.0

9. **Following are adjuant haematinics except :** **UPSC 1985**
A. Copper B. Cobalt
C. Pyridoxine D. Thiamine

10. **When neurological complications are present dose of Vitamin-B_{12} in its deficiency states is ______ microgram/d :** **DNB 2002**
A. 30-100 B. 200-300
C. 300-500 D. 500-1000

11. **Which of the following is not true about response to Vit. B_{12} in its deficiency states :** **DNB 2000**
A. Mucosal lesions heal in 1-2 weeks
B. Platelet count normalises in 10 days
C. WBC count normalises in 2-3 weeks
D. Reticocyte count starts rising after 3-4 weeks

12. **Therapeutic dose of folic acid is _____ mg/d :** **PGI 1986, 2003**
A. 1-2 B. 2-5
C. 5-10 D. 15-20

13. **Molecular weight of erythropoietin is :** **Delhi 1997, 2002**
A. 21000 B. 28000
C. 34000 D. 39000

14. **Half life of recombinant human erythropoitin is ______ hour :** **AIIMS 1999, 2004**
A. 1-5 B. 6-10
C. 10-14 D. 18-22

15. **Primary indication of erythropoitin in anemia is due to :** **AIIMS 2003**
A. Cancer chemotherapy B. AIDS
C. Chronic infections D. CRF

16. **Following are side effects of Erythropoietin except :** **PGI 1986, 1991**
A. Increased clot formation B. Hypertension
C. Allergic reaction D. Seizures

17. **Which of the following vitamin-K is produced by bacteria ?** **AIIMS 1996**
A. K_1 B. K_2
C. K_3-Menandione D. K_3-Acetomenaphthone

Ans. **8. B** **9. D** **10. D** **11. D** **12. B** **13. C**
14. B **15. D** **16. C** **17. B**

18. To reverse the effect of oral anticoagulants the preparation of choice is : DNB 1997, 99

A Phytomenadione B. Menandione
C. Ethamsylate D. Manaquinones

19. Rapid intravenous injection of emulsified vitamin-K can lead to following toxic effects : AIIMS 1991

A. Breathlessness B. A sense of constriction in chest
C. Hypertension D. Flushing

20. The dose of antihemophilic factor is ______ U/Kg : AIIMS 1993, 97

A. 1-5 B. 5-10
C. 10-15 D. 15-20

21. Following are styptics except : CSE 2002

A. Russels Viper venon B. Tannic acid
C. 1% Adrenaline D. Polidocanol

22. Streptokinase is not used if it has been used previously within _____ weeks : PGI 1997, AIIMS 2001

A. 2 B 4
C. 12 D. 24

23. Following drugs increases the effect of anticoagulants except : AIIMS 1995, 99; Delhi 1985, 90, 2001

A. Tetracycline B. Griseofulvin
C. Thyroxine D. Diphenhydramine

24. Vitamin-K increases the effect of following factors except : UPSC 1994, 2002

A. VII B. VIII
C. IX D. X

25. Duration of effect of Dicoumarol is _____ days : AIIMS 1995

A. 1-2 B. 3-7
C. 7-10 D. 10-15

26. In heparin use, which blood test is used for controlling its dosage : Orissa 1993, 99

A. BT B. CT
C. PT D. All of the above

27. Which of the following drug may be used as an antidote for heparin : TN 1993

A. Vitamin-K B. Hexadimethrine
C. Prothrombin D. None of the above

Ans. **18. A** **19. C** **20. B** **21. D** **22. D** **23. B**
24. B **25. B** **26. B** **27. B**

28. Following drugs cause both leucopenia and agranulocytosis except : AIIMS 1999, 2003

A. Thiouracil B. Streptomycin
C. Procainamide D. Lithium

29. Hemolytic reactions may be caused by following drugs except : DNB 1999; AIIMS 1996

A. Primaquine B. Nitrofurantoin
C. Methyldopa D. Meprobamate

30. Drugs to be avoided in G-6-P-D deficiency are following except : AIIMS 1989, 97, 99; UPSC 2003

A. Dapsone B. Diphenhydramine
C. Phenacetin D. Valproic acid

31. 'Koala Bear' facies may be produced by following foetal teratogen : AIIMS 1990

A. Iso-tretinoin B. Ergometrine
C. Phenytoin D. Warfarin

32. Who gave the name of the 'heparin' : AIIMS 1991

A. McLean B. Watson
C. Howett and Holt D. John and Smith

33. Half life of heparin is shorter in patients with : PGI 1996, 99

A. Cirrhosis B. Kidney failure
C. Pulmonary embolism D. None of the above

34. Danaparoid is a preparation containing heparin sulfate is used in cases of heparin induced thrombocytopenia, is obtained from gut mucosa of : DNB 1991, 98

A. Rabbit B. Rat
C. Pig D. Monkey

35. Which of the following heparinoid is obtained from Malayan pit viper venom : AIIMS 2001

A. Heparan B. Lepirudin
C. Ancrod D. Protamine

36. Which of the following oral anticoagulant has the shortest half life : AIIMS 2001

A. Phenindione B. Ethylbiscoumacetate
C. Acenocoumarol D. Bishydroxycoumarin

37. Agranulocytosis is an important side effect of : AIIMS 1992, 95

A. Phenindione B. Warfarin
C. Acenocoumarol D. Heparin

Ans. **28. D** **29. D** **30. D** **31. D** **32. C** **33. C**
34. C **35. C** **36. C** **37. A**

38. For every 200 units of heparin the dose of protamine sulphate required is _____ mg : AIIMS 1994, 95

A. 1
B. 2
C. 3
D. 4

39. After giving warfarin, the factor whose level falls first is : DNB 1997

A. VII
B. VIII
C. IX
D. X

40. Which of the following factor has the longest half life : AIIMS 1999

A. Prothrombin
B. VII
C. IX
D. X

41. The synthesis of coagulation factors diminishes within _______hour of warfarin administration : PGI 1986

A. 1-2
B. 2-4
C. 4-6
D. 10-12

42. Following factors increase the effect of anticoagulants except : AIIMS 1993, 95; DNB 1999

A. Malabsorption
B. Chronic alcoholism
C. Hypothyroidism
D. Newborns

43. Following drugs increase the anticoagulant action of warfarin except : AIIMS 1990, 95; Delhi 1996, 99, 2006

A. Cefamandole
B. Moxabactam
C. Griseofulvin
D. Celecoxib

44. Duration of action of heparin is ______ hours : UPSC 1995, 2000; Delhi 1998

A. 2-4
B. 4-6
C. 6-8
D. 8-10

45. Streptokinase is obtained from beta hemolytic streptococci group : AIIMS 2001

A. A
B. B
C. C
D. D

46. Epsilon amino-caproic acid (EACA) is an analogue of amino acid : AIIMS 2000

A. Methionine
B. Leucine
C. Isoleucine
D. Lysine

47. Rapid Intravenous injection of EACA may result in following : DNB 2001

A. Hypotension
B. Arrythmias
C. Myopathy
D. Impaired hepatic function

Ans. **38. B** **39. A** **40. A** **41. B** **42. C** **43. C**
44. B **45. C** **46. D** **47. D**

48. Aprotinin has inhibitory action on trypsin, chymotrypsin, kallikerin, plasmin, has a half life of _____ hours : PGI 2001

A. 2 B. 4
C. 6 D. 8

49. Clopidogrel in comparison to aspirin has the following differences except : AIIMS 1999, 2003

A. Higher frequency of neutropenia
B. Lower frequency of thrombocytopenia
C. Lower annual risk of primary ischemic events
D. Epigastric pain

50. Peak antiplatelet effect of ticlopidine therapy is produced after ______ days therapy : DNB 1999

A. 2-4 B. 4-6
C. 6-8 D. 8-10

51. Half life of Abciximab is ______ min :

A. 10-30 B. 30-50
C. 60-80 D. 80-100

52. Dextran-70 expands plasma volume for nearly _____ hours : CSE 1999, 2001

A. 12 B. 24
C. 36 D. 48

53. Polygeline is a polypeptide with average molecular weight of : DNB 1994, 99

A. 20,000 B. 30,000
C. 40000 D. 50000

54. Total dose of Dextran-40 should not exceed _____ml/kg in 24 hours : AIIMS 2002

A. 5 B. 10
C. 20 D. 30

55. 100 ml of blood loss means loss of ________mg elemental iron : AIIMS 1994; UPSC 1994, 2005

A. 15 B. 25
C. 50 D. 75

Ans. 48. A 49. A 50. D 51. A 52. B 53. C 54. C 55. C

EXPLANATIONS OF PHARMACOLOGICAL ASPECTS

1. Ans.— B. 3.5
2. Ans.— D. Colloidal ferric hydroxide
3. Ans.— C. About 20% excreted in urine
4. Ans.— C. Constipation
5. Ans.— B. 2-4
6. Ans.— C. Alkalosis
7. Ans.— C. 50
8. Ans.— B. 0.1
9. Ans.— D. Thiamine
10. Ans.— D. 500-1000
11. Ans.— D. Reticocyte count starts rising after 3-4 weeks
12. Ans.— B. 2-5
13. Ans.— C. 34000
14. Ans.— B. 6-10
15. Ans.— D. CRF
16. Ans.— C. Allergic reaction
17. Ans.— B. K_2
18. Ans.— A. Phytomenadione
19. Ans.— C. Hypertension
20. Ans.— B. 5-10
21. Ans.— D. Polidocanol
22. Ans.— D. 24
23. Ans.— B. Griseofulvin
24. Ans.— B. VIII

25. Ans.— B. 3-7
26. Ans.— B. CT
27. Ans.— B. Hexadimethrine
28. Ans.— D. Lithium
29. Ans.— D. Meprobamate
30. Ans.— D. Valproic acid
31. Ans.— D. Warfarin
32. Ans.— C. Howett and Holt
33. Ans.— C. Pulmonary embolism
34. Ans.— C. Pig
35. Ans.— C. Ancrod
36. Ans.— C. Acenocoumarol
37. Ans.— A. Phenindione
38. Ans.— B. 2
39. Ans.— A. VII
40. Ans.— A. Prothrombin
41. Ans.— B. 2-4
42. Ans.— C. Hypothyroidism
43. Ans.— C. Griseofulvin
44. Ans.— B. 4-6
45. Ans.— C. C
46. Ans.— D. Lysine
47. Ans.— D. Impaired hepatic function
48. Ans.— A. 2
49. Ans.— A. Higher frequency of neutropenia
50. Ans.— D. 8-10
51. Ans.— A. 10-30
52. Ans.— B. 24
53. Ans.— C. 40000
54. Ans.— C. 20
55. Ans.— C. 50

PATHOLOGICAL ASPECTS

IMPORTANT TEXT FOR PATHOLOGICAL ASPECTS

CAUSES OF MEGALOBLASTIC ANEMIA

Vitamin B12 Deficiency

Decreased intake	Inadequate diet
	Impaired absorption
	Intrinsic factor deficiency
	Pernicious anemia
	Gastrectomy
	Malabsorption states
	Diffuse intestinal disease-lymphoma, scleroderma, etc.
	Ileal resection, ileitis
	Competitive parasitic uptake
	Fish tapeworm infection
	Bacterial overgrowth in blind loops and diverticula of bowel.
Increased requirement	Pregnancy, hyperthyroidism, disseminated cancer

Folic Acid Deficiency

Decreased intake	Inadequate diet-alcoholism, infancy
	Impaired absorption
	Malabsorption states
	Intrinsic intestinal disease
	Anticonvulsants, oral contraceptives
	Hemodialysis
Increased requirement	Pregnancy, infancy, disseminated cancer, markedly increased hematopoiesis
Blocked activation	Folic acid antagonists

Unresponsive to Vitamin-B12 or Folic Acid Therapy

Metabolic inhibitors e.g. mercaptopurines, fluorouracil, cytosine etc.

Pyridoxine and thiamin-responsive megaloblastic anemia

Erythremic myelosis (Di Guglielmo's syndrome)

CLASSIFICATION OF THE LEUKEMIAS

Lymphocytic Acute (Lymphoblastic) (ALL)

L1 Small cells predominate but may vary, with some cells up to twice the diameter of the small lymphocytes. Nuclei are generally round and regular with occasional clefts. Nucleoli are often not visible. Cytoplasm is scanty. The cell population is homogeneous.

L2 Cells are heterogeneous in size and share in the features of both L1 and L3. Nuclei often show clefts. Nucleoli are often present.

L3 There is a homogenous population of large cells (3 to 4 times the diameter of small lymphocytes). Nuclei are round to oval with prominent nucleoli. Cytoplasm is abundant and deeply basophilic.

Chronic Lymphocytic (CLL).

Cells comprise a homogenous population of small mature lymphocytes, often associated with lymphocytic, well differentiated lymphoma.

Acute Myelocytic (Myeloblastic) (AML)

M1 Myeloblastic leukemia without maturation-cells are dominantly blasts without Auer rods or granules

M2 Myeloblastic leukemia with maturation—Many blasts but some maturation to promyelocytes or beyond.

M3 Hypergranular promyelocytic leukemia—Mostly promyelocytes with cytoplasm packed with peroxidase-positive granules. Many Auer rods.

M4 Myelomonocytic leukemia—Both myeloid and morocytic differentiation. Myeloid element resembles M2

M5 Monocytic leukemia—Both "monoblasts" and monocytes, the former having large round nuclei with lacy chromatin and prominent nucleoli. Diagnosis must be confirmed by fluoride-inhibited esterase reaction.

M6. Erythroleukemia—Erythropoietic elements comprise more than 50% of cells in marrow and have bizarre multilobate nuclei. May also be present in circulating blood, along with an admixture of myeloblasts and promyelocytes.

Chronic Myelocytic (CML)

Mostly neutrophils with scattered myelocytes and promyelocytes.

Acute Monocytic (included as M4, myelomonocytic leukemia)

Chronic Monocytic

Very uncommon. Mostly mature monocytes with scattered blasts. Some cells are peroxidase positive.

Special Rare Types

Histiocytic leukemia—May occur in histiocytic lymphoma.

Hairy-cell leukemia associated with leukemic reticuloendotheliosis—Of uncertain cell type. May be a B-cell or possibly a histiocyte.

Leukemia associated with Sezary's syndrome. Thought to be of T-cell origin.

Stem cell leukemia—Cells so immature as to be unidentifiable.

DIFFERENCES BETWEEN THROMBOSIS AND COAGULATION

	Thrombosis	*Coagulation*
1.	Intravascular	Extravascular
2.	Essentially a platelets deposition	A conversion of fibrinogen into fibrin
3.	Thromboplastin not essential	Essential
4.	Occurs in streaming blood	In stagnant blood
5.	Firmly attached to vessel	Weakly attached
6.	Fibrin threads and cellular components produce laminar lines of zahn	Homogenous Non-laminated
7.	Friable	Rubbery
8.	Embolism common	Rare

DIFFERENTIAL DIAGNOSIS OF MICROCYTIC HYPOCHROMIC ANEMIAS

	Serum Value	*Iron deficiency*	*Sideroblastic*	*Beta thallasemia*	*Anaemia of chronic disease*
1.	Iron	D	I	N	D
2.	Total iron binding capacity	I	N	N	D
3.	Ferritin	D	I	N	I
4.	HbA	D	D	I	N

* D—Decreased, I—Increased, N—Normal

THE NORMAL RED CELL VALUES

	Red cells	*Hb.*	*P.C.V. (Haematocrit value)*
Men	4.5-6.5 mill/cu. mm.	13.5-18.0 gm%	40 - 54%
Women	3.9 - 5.6 mill/cu. mm.	11.5-16.5 gm%	35 - 47%
Infants	4.0 - 5.6 mill/cu. mm. (full term cord blood)	13.6 - 19.6 gm%	44 - 62%
Children (1 yr.)	3.6-5.0 mill/cu. mm.	11 - 13 gm%	36 - 44%
Children (10-12 yrs.)	4.2 - 5.2 mill/cu. mm.	11.5 - 14.8 gm%	37 - 44%

MCQ'S FOR PATHOLOGICAL ASPECTS

1. FAB L_3 refers to : **AI 2007**

A. Pre B ALL
B. T-cell ALL
C. B-cell ALL
D. Mixed ALL

2. Acid phosphatase is specific for : **AIIMS 2006**

A. Monocytes
B. Myelocytes
C. B-cells
D. T-cells

3. Which of the following statements pertain to leukemia is correct ? **AI 2005**

A. Blasts of acute myeloid leukemia are typically Sudan black negative.
B. Blasts of acute lymphoblastic leukemia are typically myeloperoxidase positive.
C. Low leucocyte alkaline phosphatase score is characteristically seen in blastic phase of chronic myeloid leukemia.
D. Tartorate resistant acid phosphatase positivity is typically seen in hairy cell leukemia.

4. A 48-year old woman was admitted with a history of weakness for two months. On examination, cervical lymph nodes were found enlarged and spleen was palpable 2 cm below the costal margin. Her hemoglobin was 10.5 g/dl, platelet count 2.7 x 109/L and total leukocyte count 40 x 109/L, which included 80% mature lymphoid cells with coarse clumped chromatin. Bone marrow revealed a nodular lymphoid infiltrate. The peripheral blood lymphoid cells were positive for CD_{19}, CD_5, CD_{20} and CD_{23} and were negative for CD_{79B} and FMC-7. The histopathological examination of the lymph node in this patient will most likely exhibit effacement of lymph node architecture by : **AI 2005**

A. A pseudofollicular pattern with proliferation centers.
B. A monomorphic lymphoid proliferation with a nodular pattern
C. A predominantly follicular pattern
D. A diffuse proliferation of medium to large lymphoid cells with high mitotic rate.

Ans. **1. C** **2. D** **3. D** **4. D**

5. **A four year old boy was admitted with a history of abdominal pain and fever for two months, maculopapular rash for ten days, and dry cough, dyspnea and wheezing for three days. On examination, liver and spleen were enlarged 4 cm and 3 cm respectively below the costal margins. His hemoglobin was 10.0 g/dl. platelet count 37 x 109/L and total leukocyte count 70 x 109/L, which included 80% eosinophils. Bone marrow examination revealed a cellular marrow comprising 45% blasts and 34% eosinophils and eosinophilic precursors. The blasts stained negative for myeloperoxidase and non-specific and CD_{20}. Which one of the following statements in not true about this disease ?AI 2005**
   A. Eosinophils are not part of the Neoplastic clone
   B. t(5:14) rearrangement may be detected in blasts
   C. Peripheral blood eosinophilia may normalize with chemotherapy
   D. Inv (16) is often detected in the blasts and the eosinophils.
6. **Which of the following statement is not true ? AI 2005**
   A. Patients with IgD myeloma may present with no evident M-spike on serum electrophoresis.
   B. A diagnosis of plasma cell leukemia can be made if circulating peripheral blood plasmablasts comprise 14% of peripheral blood white cells in a patient with white blood cell count of 1 x 109/L and platelet count of 88 x 109/L.
   C. In smoldering myeloma, plasma cells constitute 10-30% of total bone marrow cellularity.
   D. In a patient with multiple myeloma, a monoclonal light chain may be detected in both serum and urine
7. **Which of the following is essential for the culmination of coagulation cascade: AI 2005**
   A. Protein-C B. Protein-S
   C. Thrombomodulin D. Thrombin
8. **Which is the most common cytogenetic abnormality in adult myelodysplastic syndrome (MDS) ? AI 2004**
   A. Trisomy 8 B. 20q-
   C. 5q- D. Monosomy 7
9. **All of the following statements about Hairy cell leukaemia are true except : AI 2004**
   A. Splenomegaly is conspicous
   B. Results from an expansion of neoplastic T lymphocytes
   C. Cells are positive for Tartarate Resistant Acid Phosphatase
   D. The cells express CD_{25} constently

Ans. **5. D** **6. B** **7. D** **8. D** **9. B**

10. The blood in the vessels normally does not clot because : AI 2004

A. Vitamin-K antagonists are present in plasma
B. Thrombin has a positive feedback on plasminogen
C. Sodium citrate in plasma chelates calcium ions
D. Vascular endothelium is smooth and coated with glycocalyx

11. A couple, with a family history of beta thalassemia major in a distant relative, has come for counselling. The husband has HbA_2 of 4.8% and the wife has HbA_2 of 2.3% The risk of having a child with beta thalassemia major is : AI 2003

A. 50% B. 25%
C. 5% D. 0%

12. Following statement about lactoferrin are true, except : AI 2003

A. It is present in secondary granules of neutrophil
B. It is present in exocrine secretions of body
C. It has great affinity for iron
D. It transports iron for erythropoiesis

13. The primary defect which leads to sickle cell anemia is : AI 2003

A. An abnormality in porphyrin part of hemoglobin
B. Replacement of glutamate by valine in β-chain of HbA
C. A nonsense mutation in the β-chain of HbA
D. Substitution of valine by glutamate in the α-chain of HbA

14. A 40 years old male had undergone splenectomy 20 years ago. Peripheral blood smear examination would show the presence of : AIIMS 2003

A. Dohle bodies B. Hypersegmented neutrophils
C. Spherocytes D. Howell-Jolly bodies

15. Prothrombin time is a function of all of the following except : TNPSC 1997

A. Factor-II B. Factor-V
C. Factor-VII D. Factor-IX

16. The sequential activation of clotting factors in Phase I of coagulation is as follows : TNPSC 1997

A. Factor-XII, Factor-VIII, Factor-XI, Factor-IX
B. Factor-XII, Factor-XI, Factor-IX, Factor -VIII
C. Factor-VIII, Factor-XII, Factor-IX , Factor-XI
D. Factor-IX, Factor-VIII, Factor-XI, Factor-XII

17. Following are the complications of blood transfusion except : NIMHANS 1997

A. DIC B. HIV
C. Pyrexia & rigors D. Hepatitis-A

Ans. **10. D** **11. D** **12. D** **13. B** **14. D** **15. D**
16. B **17. D**

18. **Correct about Erythropoietin is following except : Kerala 1991**
A. Is a glycoprotein
B. Has been isolated in pure form
C. Is produced mainly by the kidney
D. Can be measured by radio-immunoassay
E. None of the above

19. **Characteristic features of the anaemia of chronic disorders include except : TN 1992**
A. Normocytic red cells
B. Low plasma iron
C. High TIBC
D. Increased iron in reticulo-endothelial cells
E. Increased plasma copper

20. **The macrophages originate from : Bihar 1991**
A. Monocytes B. Tissue cells
C. Giant cells D. Lymphocytes
E. Foreign body

21. **Plasma cells are increased in : AMU 1986**
A. Rheumatoid arthritis B. Acute appendicitis
C. Leukaemia D. Bronchitis
E. Bristles of burnt skin

22. **Spherocytes are seen in peripheral smear in following except: Kerala 1997**
A. Hereditary spherocytosis B. Hereditary ellipcytosis
C. Hemolytic anaemia D. Sickle cell anaemia

23. **Acute leukaemia may be caused by exposure to : JIPMER 1998**
A. Benzene B. Vinyl chloride
C. Nickel D. Naphthylamine

24. **First Hb to appear in foetal life : MP 1998**
A. HbA_2 B. HbF
C. HbA D. Gower Hb

25. **The activated partial thromboplastin time test is useful for the detection of deficiency of following except : DNB 1990**
A. Factor-XI B. High molecular weight kininogen
C. Pre-kallikrein D. Factor-VII
E. Factor-XII

26. **Elevated levels of alkaline phosphatase are typical of the following except : AMU 1986, 93**
A. Cirrhosis B. Obstructive jaundice
C. Myocardial infarction D. Polycythemia vera

Ans. 18. E 19. C 20. A 21. A 22. D 23. A
24. B 25. D 26. C

27. Hypersegmented polymorph is characteristically seen in : Rohtak 1987, 96

A. Infections
B. Iron deficiency
C. Folic acid deficiency
D. Malignancy

28. Approximately what percentage of transferrin is saturated with iron in the serum of a normal individual : DNB 1989, 95

A. 10%
B. 33%
C. 50%
D. 66%

29. The colour of hemosiderin is : AP 1991

A. Black
B. Golden yellow
C. Greenish
D. Red

30. The total leucocyte count in acute myeloblastic leukaemia is : DNB 1984, 91

A. 5,000-10,000
B. 20,000-25,000
C. 45,000-50,000
D. Above 1,00,000

31. Coomb's positive hemolysis is seen in : PGI 1997

A. ITP
B. SLE
C. TTP
D. Dapsone intake

32. Life span of neutrophil is : PGI 1977

A. 6 hours
B. 6 days
C. 10 days
D. 15 days

33. Chromosomal abnormality seen in promyelocytic leukaemia is : PGI 1985, 92

A. 17-15t
B. 21-9t
C. 22-9t
D. None

34. Bone marrow infilteration is seen with the following except : Punjab 1997

A. Retinoblastoma
B. Neuroblastoma
C. Non-Hodgkin's lymphoma
D. Wilm's tumour

35. Triad of gross hematuria, pain and abdominal mass in renal cell carcinoma is present in : NIMHANS 1986, 94

A. 10%
B. 30%
C. 40%
D. 60%

36. Gower Type-I Hb is : DNB 1991

A. Alpha 2 delta 2
B. Epsilon 2 Delta-2
C. Alpha 2 gamma 2
D. Epsilon 2 gamma 2

Ans. **27. C** **28. B** **29. B** **30. B** **31. B** **32. C**
33. A **34. C** **35. A** **36. B**

37. **In idiopathic thrombocytopaenic purpura : Delhi 1983, 96**
A. Increase of megakaryocytes in marrow
B. Decrease of megakaryocytes in marrow
C. Increase of platelets in blood
D. None of the above

38. **Of the following, the earliest step in the formation of a thrombus is : AI 1990**
A. Formation of fibrin
B. Trapping of erythrocytes
C. Adherance of platelets to vascular intima
D. Activation of Hageman's factor

39. **The normal percentage of reticulocyte count in adult is : Rohtak 1986, 93**
A. 5 to 6 B. 0.2 to 2
C. 7 to 10 D. None of the above

40. **Confirmation of myelofibrosis is by : JIPMER 1986, 97**
A. Bone marrow aspiration
B. Peripheral smear
C. Leukocytes alkaline phosphatase in neutrophils
D. Bone marrow biopsy

41. **The best suited anticoagulant for osmotic fragility test is : AIIMS 1986, 91**
A. Heparin B. EDTA
C. Trisodium citrate D. Potassium oxalate

42. **Vitamin-K deficiency is seen in : AIIMS 1988, 93**
A. Hepatic jaundice B. Prehepatic jaundice
C. Obstructive jaundice D. All of the above

43. **In myelodysplatic syndrome the following is characteristically seen in peripheral smear : DNB 1989, 98**
A. Acanthocyte B. Stomatocyte
C. Tear drop cell D. Helmet cell

44. **The electrophoresis method is commonly employed for assessing : DNB 1991**
A. Snake and spider bites
B. Iron deficiency anaemia
C. Haemoglobinopathies
D. Haemolytic uraemic syndrome

45. **The normal total iron binding capacity is : UPSC 1988, 93**
A. 0.5-1.0 mg/litre B. 1.5-2.5 mg/litre
C. 1.0-1.5 mg/litre D. 2.5-4 mg/litre

Ans. 37. A 38. C 39. B 40. D 41. D 42. C
43. C 44. C 45. D

46. All of these are dietary sources of Iron except : UPSC 1986, 96

A. Liver B. Kidney
C. Egg yolk D. Milk

47. Hypersplenism is associated with all these conditions except : UPSC 1986, 91

A. Cirrhosis liver (Banti's syndrome)
B. Fatty's syndrome
C. Long standing sickle cell anaemia
D. Gaucher's disease

48. Response to iron in iron deficiency anemia is denoted by : Delhi 1993

A. Restoration of enzymes
B. Reticulocytosis
C. Increase in iron binding capacity
D. Increase in hemoglobin

49. Megaloblastic anemia in pregnancy is treated with vitamin : Delhi 1988, 93

A. B_1 B. B_2
C. Folic acid D. B_{12}

50. Bone marrow contain lymphocytes in following except : AI 1993

A. Kala Azar
B. Hypoplastic anemia
C. Acute Myeloid leukemia
D. Chronic myeloid leukemia

51. Which is not true of Platelet transfusions? JIPMER 1990, 92

A. Platelets are effective for 9-10 days
B. Is effective in ITP
C. Effect decreases with repeated usage
D. Are used in DIC

52. Following are present in Pernicious anemia except : JIPMER 1992

A. Antibodies to Vit. B_{12}
B. Antibodies to intrinsic factor
C. Decreased absorption of Vit. B_{12}
D. Antibodies to parietal cell

53. Leukoerythroblastic reaction is seen in following except : JIPMER 1992

A. Secondaries in bone B. Multiple myeloma
C. Hemolytic anemia D. Lymphoma

Ans. **46. D** **47. C** **48. B** **49. C** **50. A** **51. A**
52. A **53. C**

54. Microcytic hypochromic anemia is seen in following except : **AI 1989; JIPMER 1992, 95**

A. PNB
B. Sickle cell anemia
C. Thalassemia
D. Iron deficiency

55. Following are features of Thrombus except : **JIPMER 1992**

A. Friable
B. Easily detached
C. Dry
D. Mottled

56. Rise in ESR occurs when there is increase in : **JIPMER 1992**

A. Leucocytes
B. Protein
C. Complements
D. Hageman factor

57. Tachyzoites are seen in : **PGI 1997**

A. Toxoplasma
B. Toxocara
C. Pulm. eosinophilia
D. Ascariasis

58. Sideroblastic anemia is seen in chronic poisoning of : **AIIMS 1992**

A. Lead
B. Arsenic
C. Copper
D. Mercury

59. All the following are true of Hereditary Spherocytosis except : **AIIMS 1992**

A. Autosomal dominant
B. Normal or decreased MCV
C. Splenomegaly
D. Haemolytic crisis is the usual presentation

60. Which of the following is a late feature of Multiple myeloma ? **AIIMS 1992**

A. M spike
B. Osteolytic lesion
C. Renal failure
D. Raised serum alkaline phosphatase

61. Leukoerythroblastic reaction is seen in all except : **Jipmer 1992**

A. Lymphoma
B. Secondaries in bone
C. Multiple myeloma
D. Hemolytic anemia

62. Which is seen in Hemolytic uremic syndrome : **AI 1992**

A. Coombs test positive
B. Thrombocytopenia
C. Hypofibrinogenemia
D. Uremia

63. The consequences of the transfusion of one litre of B-positive blood into an O +ve recipient are likely to include all the following except : **Manipal 1994**

A. Blockage of the pulmonary artery by agglutinated cells
B. Haemolysis
C. Oliguria/anuria
D. Pyrexia

Ans. **54. B** **55. B** **56. B** **57. A** **58. A** **59. D**
60. C **61. D** **62. C** **63. A**

64. Which is not associated with sickle cell anemia : AI 1992

A. Ankle ulcer B. Cardiomegaly
C. Leucopenia D. Fish mouth vertebra

65. Pre-existing antibodies in renal transplantation leads to : AI 1992

A. Hyperacute rejection B. Acute Rejection
C. Chronic rejection D. Graft Vs Host Reaction

66. In thromboasthenia, there is a defect in : JIPMER 1991

A. Platelet aggregation
B. Platelet adhesion
C. Decreased ADP release
D. Disordered platelet secretion

67. Leucocytosis is seen in following except : JIPMER 1991

A. Brucellosis B. Acute MI
C. Typhoid D. Diphtheria

68. CML is characterised by following except : JIPMER 1991

A. Leukocytosis
B. Thrombocytosis
C. Increased leukocyte alkaline phosphatase
D. Increased serum vitamin B-12

69. Dithionite test is done for assessing : AMU 1984, 90

A. HbF B. HbE
C. HbA D. HbC
E. HbS

70. All the following statements about neutrophil granulocytes are true except : Manipal 1994

A. They are motile
B. They cannot leave the circulation
C. They contain lysosomes
D. They are attracted chemically to sites of inflammation

71. The average specific gravity of whole blood is : PGI 1980, 85, 93

A. 1.010 B. 1.035
C. 1.055 D. 1.090

72. Peripheral smear of Sickle cell anemia patient may show : AIIMS 1986, 92

A. Howell Jolly bodies B. Reticulocytsis
C. Ovalocytosis D. All of the above

73. Antischkow myocyte is a : DNB 1994

A. Basophil B. Lymphocyte
C. Histiocyte D. Neutrophil

Ans. 64. C 65. A 66. A 67. C 68. C 69. E
70. B 71. C 72. D 73. B

74. For whole blood transfusion which of the following is the indication of : PGI 1982, 94

A. Acute blood loss
B. Anemia
C. Chronic granulocytic leukaemia
D. Thrombocytopenic purpura

75. The fungus which causes the vascular lesion with thrombus formation : AIIMS 1982

A. Coccidiodomycosis
B. Mucormycosis
C. Histoplasmosis
D. Blastomycosis

76. For exchange transfusion in haemolytic disease of the new born : AIIMS 1982, 93

A. Fresh blood should be used
B. Only plasma should be used
C. Old blood of 7 days duration can be used
D. All of the above can be used

77. Chronic haemoglobinuria can be caused by : AIIMS 1981,92

A. Incompatible blood transfusion
B. Paroxysmal cold haemoglobinuria
C. Paroxysmal nocturnal haemoglobinuria
D. Exertional haemoglobinuria

78. Granules of eosinophils contain all of the following except : PGI 1982,94

A. Histaminase
B. Phospholipase
C. Aryl sulphatase-B
D. Trypsin

79. Occlusive arterial thrombi are most frequently encountered in : AIIMS 1982, 95

A. Cerebral arteries
B. Coronary arteries
C. Femoral arteries
D. Renal arteries

80. Sickle cell anaemia is frequently associated with all of the following except : AIIMS 1983, 99

A. Fatty change in heart
B. Nephrosis
C. Cholelithiasis
D. Hyperplastic bone marrow

81. The replacement of red marrow by fatty marrow in bony cavities starts at the age of : AIIMS 1983, 92

A. 1-3 years
B. 4-5 years
C. 6-9 years
D. 9-12 years

Ans. **74. A** **75. B** **76. A** **77. C** **78. D** **79. B**
80. B **81. B**

82. Hageman factor in clotting is : PGI 1986, 93

A. Factor-III B. Factor-VII
C. Factor-XII D. Factor-VIII

83. If from a finger prick blood has to be drawn for both WBC and RBC counts, suck blood for WBC count first because : AIIMS 1985, 91

A. WBC's would be less in the latter drops
B. Large quantity is required for WBC count
C. RBC's are more in the first few drops
D. None of the above

84. A false positive sickling test may be found in : AIIMS 1980, 92

A. Recently transfused blood
B. Infected blood sample
C. HbC-Harlem
D. All of the above

85. Mild hemolytic anaemia is associated with vitamin——— deficiency : AIIMS 1983, 98

A. B1 B. E
C. A D. C

86. Lines of Zahn occur in : AI 1990

A. Postmortem clot B. Infarct
C. Embolus D. Coralline thrombus

87. In a patient with chronic lymphocytic leukaemia, which of the following findings is least likely in the peripheral blood smear ? Manipal 1994

A. Essentially normal platelet distribution
B. Numerous lymphoblasts
C. Numerous mature lymphocytes
D. Numerous smudge cells

88. The normal adult blood contains : AIIMS 1986, 92

A. Only HbA B. HbA + HbA
C. HbA + HbF D. HbA + HbF + HbA2

89. Bleeding diathesis is a common presenting symptom in : PGI 1982, 90

A. Acute promyelocytic Leukaemia
B. Chronic myeloid Leukaemia
C. Myelomonocytic Leukaemia
D. Chronic Lymphoid Leukaemia

90. "Kleihauer test" is used to know : UPSC 1988, 93

A. Number of foetal cells in maternal circulation
B. To find out the deficiency of factor-VIII
C. To find out the exact number of platelets
D. None of the above

Ans. **82. C** **83. B** **84. D** **85. B** **86. D** **87. B** **88. D** **89. A** **90. A**

91. Which of the following is not a feature of the anti-mortem thrombus : AIIMS 1980, 92

A. They are firmly attached to the vessel wall
B. They are homogenous, non-laminated
C. They are friable
D. Variegated colouration is present

92. Which of the following are the complications of bone marrow transplantation : AIIMS 1984, 93

A. Graft rejection B. Graft vs. host disease
C. Severe infection D. All of the above

93. Blood when stored at 4°C can be kept for : AIIMS 1984, 91

A. 7 days B. 14 days
C. 21 days D. 28 days

94. Palpable purpura is seen in following except : AIIMS 1990

A. Idiopathic thrombocytopenic purpura
B. Drug induced
C. Mixed essential cryoglobulinemia
D. Vasculitis

95. Spherocytosis in peripheral blood is not found in : AIIMS 1988, 93

A. Thalassemia major
B. Hereditary spherocytosis
C. G-6-P-D deficiency
D. Autoimmune hemolytic anaemia

96. Blast cells in acute lymphoblastic leukemia can be diagnosed by : AIIMS 1983, 88, 96

A. Sudan black
B. Acid phosphatase
C. Leucocytic alkaline phosphatase
D. Cholinesterase

97. Findings of intravascular hemolysis are except : PGI 1987, 91

A. Increased hemoglobulinuria
B. Increased hemosiderinuria
C. Increased haptoglobulins
D. Hemoglobinemia

98. ESR depends on : PGI 1987, 92

A. Viscosity B. Fibrinogen
C. Rouleaux formation D. Verticality of tube
E. All of the above

Ans. 91. B 92. D 93. C 94. A 95. C 96. A
97. C 98. E

99. **Histocytosis is a prominent feature in :** **Delhi 1986, 95**
A. Cardiac haemolytic anemia
B. Severe burns injury
C. Microangiopathic haemolytic anemia
D. All of the above

100. **Test of Hess is done to assess :** **Delhi 1983, 93**
A. Bleeding time
B. Capillary fragility
C. Clotting time
D. Prothrombin time

101. **The Myeloproliferative Syndrome of Demeashak includes all of the following except :** **AIIMS 1986, 90**
A. Angiogenic myeloid metaplasia
B. Thrombocythemia
C. Erythroleukemia
D. Megaloblastic hyperplasia

102. **Which of the following laboratory findings is not characteristic of idiopathic thrombocytopenia purpura ?** **Manipal 1994**
A. Normal leucocyte count
B. Normal prothrombin time, partial thromboplastin time and thrombin time
C. Platelet count <50,000/mm^3
D. Decreased number of megakaryocytes in the bone marrow

103. **Pancytopenia is associated with :** **AIIMS 1988, 91**
A. Paroxysmal nocturnal hemoglobinuria
B. Paroxysmal cold hemoglobulinuria
C. Thalassemia
D. Hereditary spherocytosis

104. **In Thalassemia, all of the following are seen except :** **AIIMS 1988, 93**
A. Target cells
B. Mongoloid facies
C. Increased osmotic fragility
D. Microcytic hypochromic anaemia

105. **Prothrombin time is increased in :** **AIIMS 1988, 96**
A. Willebrand's disease
B. Afibrinogenemia
C. Qualitative defect of platelets
D. Thrombocytopenia

Ans. 99. D 100. B 101. A 102. D 103. A 104. C 105. A

106. Which of the following is not useful in asbestosis : **AIIMS 1987; UPSC 1986, 91**

A. Serum ferritin
B. Stool for ova
C. Stool for occult blood
D. Bone marrow examination

107. IgM spike is usually seen in : **AIIMS 1987, 93**

A. Thymoma
B. Lymphoblastic leukaemia
C. Macroglobulinemia
D. α-chain disease

108. The indirect antiglobulin (Coombs') test is used to : **Manipal 1995**

A. Confirm antibacterial antibodies in the serum
B. Determine delayed hypersensitivity reactions
C. Detect "incomplete" antibody in the serum
D. Detect red blood cells coated by globulin in vivo

109. True about idiopathic thrombocytopenic purpura : **AIIMS 1987, 92**

A. It is diagnosed by poor clot retraction
B. Splenomegaly is present in a majority
C. Remits of its own without any treatment in all
D. Decrease in megakaryocytes in bone marrow

110. In a normal person, which of the following statement is correct regarding distribution of platelets in the body : **PGI 1990**

A. 70% circulating and 30% in splenic pool
B. 30% circulating and 70% in splenic pool
C. 50% circulating and 50% in splenic pool
D. All the platelets circulates in the peripheral blood

111. Sezary-Lutzner cells are found in : **AIIMS 1987, 92**

A. Burkitt's lymphoma
B. Hodgkin's lymphoma
C. Non-Hodgkin's lymphoma
D. Mycosis fungoides

112. Impaired platelet function is seen in following except: **AIIMS 1990**

A. Von Willebrand's disease
B. Cryoglobulinemia
C. Multiple myeloma
D. Idiopathic thrombocytopenic purpura

113. All of the following are needed for clotting except : **AIIMS 1990**

A. Calcium
B. Collagen
C. Platelets
D. Local stasis

Ans. **106. C** **107. C** **108. C** **109. A** **110. A** **111. D**
112. D **113. D**

114. Majority of chronic lymphocytic leukaemia is of ______ type: **PGI 1986, 93**

A. T-cell
B. B-cell
C. Null cell
D. Mixed B-cell and T-cell

115. In a patient with hemolytic anaemia, the following change is seen : **PGI 1986, 91**

A. Serum bilirubin more than 15 mg/dl
B. Increase in Urine haemosiderin
C. Increase in Serum haptoglobulin
D. None of the above

116. Rewarmed blood may be kept prior to use for : **PGI 1989, 95**

A. 3 minutes
B. 30 minutes
C. 3 hours
D. All are wrong

117. In polycythaemia vera, it is usual to find : **Manipal 1996**

A. Defective haemostasis
B. Megaloblastic erythropoeisis
C. Reduced leucocyte alkaline phosphatase
D. Reduced serum vitamin-B_{12} content

118. Which of the following statements about acute lymphoblastic leukaemia (ALL) is true ? **Manipal 1996**

A. B-cell ALL has the best prognosis
B. Girls are more often affected than boys
C. Stained blood films commonly show Auer rods
D. Widespread lymph node enlargement may occur

119. Secondary polycythemia is characteristically seen in: **Delhi 1986, 93**

A. Miliary tuberculosis
B. Carcinomatosis
C. Hypernephroma
D. Chronic bronchitis with airway obstruction

120. Normocytic normochromic anaemia is seen in : **Delhi 1986, 95**

A. Hypoplastic anaemia
B. Hypothyroidism
C. Chronic blood loss
D. Ankylostomiasis

121. Deficiency of B-lymphocytes is detected by : **Delhi 1986, 97**

A. Patch test
B. Decrease Immunoglobulins
C. Graft rejection
D. Total leucocytic count

122. Vasculitis is seen in : **Delhi 1986, 92**

A. Sickle cell anaemia
B. Thalassemia
C. SLE
D. Amniotic fluid embolism

Ans. **114. B** **115. D** **116. B** **117. A** **118. D** **119. C** **120. B** **121. B** **122. C**

123. Acute myelogenous leukemia is cytochemically : AIIMS 1986, 92

A. Peroxidase negative B. ANE positive
C. NCE positive D. Sudan Black B-negative

124. Tissue and blood eosinophilia is seen in infestation with : AIIMS 1987; Delhi 1986, 87, 91

A. Ascaris B. Echinococcus
C. Enterobius D. Trichinella

125. In Virchow's triad for thrombosis, which of the following is not included: Delhi 1987, 95

A. Stasis
B. Inflammation in blood vessel
C. Change in blood composition (shape of cell etc.)
D. Hypoproteinemia

126. Philadelphia chromosome is an example of : CSE 1998

A. Balanced translocation
B. Deletion
C. Non-dysjunction
D. Duplication

127. Common site of haemopoiesis in foetus is : Delhi 1984, 89, 94

A. Liver B. Spleen
C. Bone marrow D. Gut

128. Commonest leukemia in bone is : DNB 1989, 93

A. CML B. CLL
C. ALL D. AML

129. Which of the following is the best source of factor-VIII? Karnataka 1998

A. Fresh blood B. Fresh frozen plasma
C. Cryoprecipitate D. Platelet concentrate

130. Karyotypic change of Acute Promyelocytic leukaemia is : Karnataka 1998

A. t 15 : 17 B. t 18 : 14
C. t 8 : 22 D. t11 : 22

131. Modified Cutler method is used to measure : DNB 1988, 92

A. BT B. CT
C. PT D. ESR

132. ESR is low in the following except : PGI 1985, 97

A. CHF B. Newborn
C. Polycythemia D. Sickle cell disease
E. Menstruation

Ans. **123. C** **124. D** **125. D** **126. A** **127. A** **128. A**
129. C **130. A** **131. D** **132. B**

133. Linzenmeter is used to measure : AIIMS 1985, 91

A. BT B. CT
C. PTT D. CRT
E. ESR

134. Replacement of red marrow by fatty marrow in bony cavities starts at the age of : AIIMS 1982, 90

A. 1-2 years B. 2-3 years
C. 4-5 years D. 6-7 years

135. The M component in multiple myeloma is frequently: Delhi 1985, 93

A. IgG B. IgM
C. IgA D. IgD

136. Auer rods (reddish, abnormal lysosomes) are usually seen in : AIIMS 1984, 97

A. Lymphocytes B. Neutrophils
C. Monocytes D. Basophilis

137. Which type of immunological reactions involve the Rh incompatibility: Bihar 1991

A. Type-I B. Type -II
C. Type-IV D. Type -V
E. Any of the above depending upon severity

138. The number of band present in thalassemia trait (Bhs) is : Bihar 1991

A. 1 B. 2
C. 3 D. 4

139. Coomb's test (direct) is positive in : Bihar 1988, 1991

A. Cold agglutinin B. Warm agglutinin
C. IgM D. IgG

140. Hemophilia -A is due to deficiency of factor : Bihar 1991, AIIMS 1990

A. VII B. VIII
C. IX D. XI
E. XII

141. Persons with sickle cell trait are partly resistant to : AIIMS 1981, 92

A. Typhoid
B. Streptococcal septicaemia
C. Viral pneumonia
D. Weil's disease
E. Malaria

Ans. **133. E** **134. C** **135. A** **136. C** **137. B** **138. B**
139. D **140. B** **141. E**

142. Immediately after a strong thermal injury vaso-constriction occurs, which usually lasts for : **Kerala 1988, 95**

A. 0 to 10 seconds
B. 30 to 60 seconds
C. 1 to 5 minutes
D. 10 to 30 minutes

143. The best investigation to establish diagnosis of thalassemia is : **AIIMS 1986, 92**

A. Osmotic fragility
B. Coomb's test
C. Hb A2 estimation
D. HbF estimation

144. Which of the following is not seen in aplastic anaemia: **AIIMS 1987, 92**

A. Anamia
B. Purpura
C. Haemorrhage
D. Splenomegaly

145. True about pernicious anaemia is : **AIIMS 1986, 93**

A. Totally cured by Vitamin-B_{12} injections in a few weeks
B. Haemosiderin is decreased in bone marrow
C. Not seen in orientalis
D. Not a cause of megaloblastic anaemia

146. The commonest immunological type of multiple myeloma is : **AIIMS 1986, 95**

A. IgG kappa light chain
B. IgA kappa light chain
C. IgD lambda light chain
D. IgM type

147. The commonest histologic type of Hodgkin's disease in India is : **AIIMS 1986, 91**

A. Lymphocytic predominance
B. Lymphocytic depletion
C. Mixed cellular type
D. Nodular sclerosing type

148. Non-Hodgkin's lymphoma involving brain is : **AIIMS 1986, 97**

A. Lymphocytic predominance
B. Small cell type
C. Eosinophilic predominance
D. Undifferentiated type

149. The commonest leukaemia in Northern India is : **AIIMS 1989, 92**

A. AML
B. CML
C. ALL
D. CLL

Ans. 142. C 143. C 144. D 145. C 146. A 147. D 148. D 149. B

150. An increase in bleeding and clotting time is seen in : AIIMS 1986, 95
A. Hemophilia
B. Christmas disease
C. Von Willebrand's disease
D. Idiopathic thrombocytopenic purpura

151. The erythropoiesis is decreased in all except: AIIMS 1987, 90
A. Sideropenia
B. Decreased iron intake
C. Thalassemia
D. Immunosuppressive intake

152. In a thrombus, first evidence of fibrosis is seen after : AIIMS 1985, 92
A. 1st week B. 2nd week
C. 3rd week D. 4th week

153. In iron deficiency anaemia true is : UPSC 1984, 86; AIIMS 1985, 94

	Serum iron	*Iron binding capacity*
A.	Low	Low
B.	High	Low
C.	Low	High
D.	Low	Normal

154. Target cell is seen in : PGI 1994
A. Thalassemia major
B. Vit-B_{12} deficiency anaemia
C. Sickle cell anaemia
D. Children

155. Reticulocytosis is not seen with : AIIMS 1994
A. Hereditary spherolytosis
B. Following acute bleeding
C. Paroxysmal nocturnal haemoglobinuria
D. Anaemia of chronic renal failure

156. Following are seen in multiple myeloma except : AIIMS 1995
A. Plasmacytosis>2% on bone marrow
B. Lytic bone lesion
C. Hypercalcemia
D. Serum alk. phosphatase activity

157. In beta thalassemia, not true is : Delhi 1995
A. HbF is 15%
B. Serum normal increased or decreased
C. Fragility of cells is increased
D. MCV and MCH are low

Ans. 150. C 151. C 152. A 153. C 154. A 155. D
156. A 157. C

158. In sickle cell anaemia, at pH 8.6 how many bands are seen on chromatography : Delhi 1995

A. 2 B. 3
C. 4 D. 5

159. In DIC, false is : AI 1995

A. PT is prolonged
B. APTT is normal
C. Fibrinogen is decreased
D. Thrombocytopenia

160. In multiple myeloma, best indicator of prognosis is : AI 1995

A. Serum β_2-microglobulins
B. No. of plasma cells in marrow
C. Level of Ca^{++}
D. None of the above

161. Intrinsic factor of Castle deficiency causes : AI 1995

A. Megaloblastic anemia B. Cooley's anemia
C. Pernicious anemia D. Aplastic anemia

162. Eosinophils are increased in following except : AP 1995

A. Hodgkin's disease B. Bronchial asthma
C. Loeffer's syndrome D. Miliary tuberculosis

163. Target cells are most commonly noted in : Rajasthan 1989, 90

A. HbAC B. HbSS
C. HbCC D. HbEE

164. Bone marrow aspiration is done to confirm all except: PGI 1988, 93

A. Niemann Pick disease B. Tay Sach disease
C. Gaucher's disease D. Mucopolysaccharidosis

165. The most common cause of iron deficiency in adults is : AIIMS 1988; PGI 1988, 93

A. Hemolysis
B. Inadequate dietary intake of meat
C. Inadequate intake of iron supplements
D. Chronic blood loss

166. Dohle bodies are characteristically seen in : Delhi 1983, 92

A. AML B. ALL
C. AMOL D. None of the above

167. On performing paper electrophoresis of pH 8.9, the fastest moving haemoglobin is : AIIMS 1984, 96

A. HbH B. Hb Bart's
C. HbS D. HbA

Ans. **158. A** **159. B** **160. A** **161. C** **162. D** **163. C**
164. B **165. D** **166. D** **167. A**

168. Waldenstrom's macroglobulinemia is characterised by all of the following except : **AIIMS 1983, 92**

A. Flame cells
B. Thesaurocytes
C. Lymphocystoid plasma cells
D. Helmet cells

169. All of the following are the causes of eosinophilia except of : **PGI 1983, 88; AMC 1986, 94**

A. Loeffer's pneumonia
B. Fungal infection
C. Tropical eosinophilia
D. ACTH intake

170. Serum does not contain : **Karnataka 1998**

A. Prothrombin
B. Calcium
C. Factor-VII
D. Factor-IX

171. Low LAP score is not found in : **PGI 1986, 95**

A. PNH
B. Aplastic anaemia
C. Infectious mononucleosis
D. CML

172. Conditions predisposing to leukemia include all except : **AIIMS 1985,93**

A. Ionising radiation
B. Myelofibrosis
C. Infectious mononucleosis
D. Polycythemia vera

173. "Extramedullary haemopoiesis" means : **AIIMS 1982, 90**

A. Haemopoiesis occur outside the medulla
B. Spleen and liver resume haemopoiesis
C. Expansion of haemopoiesis down the long bones
D. None of the above

174. Which of the following is the best single indicator of bone marrow iron reserves ? **AIIMS 1984, 92**

A. Serum iron
B. Serum ferritin concentration
C. Haemoglobin
D. Serum transferrin level

175. Haemolytic anemia does not result from : **PGI 1983, 94**

A. Congenital spherocytosis
B. Sickle cell disease
C. Thalassemic haemosiderosis
D. Erythroblastosis foetalis

Ans. 168. D 169. D 170. C 171. C 172. C 173. B
174. B 175. C

176. Bone marrow aspiration is contraindicated in : Delhi 1983, 96

A. Hepatic cellular disease
B. Cor pulmonale
C. Acute leukaemia
D. Haemophilia

177. Which does not cause disseminated intravascular coagulation ? PGI 1986; AI 1989, 94

A. Snake bite B. Malaria
C. Hemophilia D. Polycythemia

178. Earliest sign of megaloblastic anaemia is : AIIMS 1985; AI 1989, 94

A. Increased MVC
B. Increased neutrophil segmentation
C. Altered ME ratio
D. Decreased hemoglobin

179. Spherocytosis is best diagnosed by : Rajasthan 1998

A. Peripheral blood smear B. BM aspiration
C. Plasma D. Splenic puncture

180. Exudation of plasma and Leucocytes in acute inflammation is from the : AIIMS 1985; PGI 1989, 93

A. Venules B. Capillaries
C. Arterioles D. Arterioles and capillaries

181. ESR is not rapid in : AIIMS 1985, 91

A. Shock
B. Menstruation
C. Congestive heart failure
D. Osteoarthritis

182. Which Hb has protective effect on sickling : AIIMS 1981, 93

A. C B. F
C. D D. E

183. The term Cooley's anemia is also used to denote : AIIMS 1981, 95

A. Hereditary spherocytosis
B. Alpha Thalassaemia
C. Beta Thalassemia major
D. Beta Thalassaemia minor

184. Direct Coomb's test is positive in hemolytic anaemia due to : AIIMS 1987, 92

A. Paroxysmal cold hemoglobinuria
B. Paroxysmal nocturnal hemoglobinuria
C. Hereditary spherocytosis
D. Idiopathic thrombocytopenic purpura

Ans. **176. D** **177. C** **178. B** **179. A** **180. B** **181. C**
182. B **183. C** **184. D**

185. Normal myeloid erythroid ratio is : **AIIMS 1985, 96**

A. 2: 1 B. 1 : 1
C. 3:1 D. 5 : 1
E. 6 : 1

186. False positive direct Coomb's test may occur in : **PGI 1986, 92**

A. Penicillin therapy B. Cephaloridine therapy
C. Phenacetin therapy D. All of the above

187. The number of haemoglobin molecules per red blood cell are : **PGI 1982, 95**

A. 2 million B. 40 million
C. 280 million D. 360 million

188. In a normal person, haemoglobin becomes———% saturated with oxygen in lungs : **PGI 1983, 99**

A. 45 B. 65
C. 95 D. 100

189. Spur cell anemia is related to : **PGI 1981**

A. Chronic liver disease B. Acute blood loss
C. Chronic blood loss D. None of the above

190. Changes seen in the islets in association with diabetes mellitus include all of the following except : **AIIMS 1980, 91**

A. Amyloidosis of the islets
B. Leukocytic infiltration of islets
C. Calcification of islets
D. Fibrosis of islets

191. Hairy cell leukemia affects : **AI 1999**

A. T. cell B. B. cell
C. Macrophage D. Monocyte

192. The type of lymphocyte which is predominant in chronic lymphocytic leukemia : **AI 1988, 94**

A. T-Lymphocyte B. B-Lymphocyte
C. K-cells D. Helper T-Lymphocytes

193. Red cell intrinsic abnormality leading to hemolytic anemia include the following except : **Karnataka 1989, 92**

A. Hereditary spherocytosis
B. Hemolytic elliptocytosis
C. Proxymal noctarnal hemoglobinuria
D. Thalassemia

Ans. **185. C** **186. D** **187. C** **188. C** **189. A** **190. C**
191. B **192. B** **193. D**

194. The type of anemia seen in chronic infections is : PGI 1993

A. Microcytic, hypochromic
B. Normocytic, hypochromic
C. Dimorphic type
D. Normocytic, normochromic

195. Increased iron binding capacity and decreased serum iron are seen in: PGI 1993

A. Anaemia of chronic infection
B. Sideroblastic anaemia
C. Thalassaemia
D. Sickle cell anemia

196. Which of the following sites is not rich in thromboplastin : PGI 1993

A. Lungs
B. Hypothalamus
C. Prostate
D. Pancreas

197. von Willebrand factor is : West Bengal 1994; JIPMER 2002

A. Platelet aggregator
B. Platelet aggregator inhibitor
C. Plasminogen activator
D. None of the above

198. The one state prothrombin time is an index of the function of : Karnataka 1994

A. Extrinsic pathway of coagulation
B. Intrinsic pathway of coagulation
C. Platelet function
D. Capillary function

199. Megaloblastic bone marrow reaction is seen in : AMU 1991

A. Idiopathic thrombocytopenic purpura
B. Sickle cell anaemia
C. Thalassaemia
D. Pernicious anaemia

200. Philadelphia chromosome (Ph1) is commonly associated with : AMU 1989, 93

A. Chronic lymphatic leukemia
B. Leukemoid reaction
C. Acute monocytic leukemia
D. None of the above

201. For determination of ESR by Western gren method, the only anticoagulant used is : DNB 1991

A. EDTA
B. Double oxalate
C. Trisodium citrate
D. Heparin

Ans. 194. D 195. B 196. B 197. A 198. A 199. D
200. D 201. C

202. Which of the following haemoglobinopathies is characterized by increased affinity for oxygen : DNB 1989, 95

A. Hb chesapeake
B. β-thalassaemia
C. HbS
D. Hb-M Boston

203. Serum Iron levels are low in which one of the following conditions : AMC 1985, 96

A. Thalassaemia major
B. Haemochromatosis
C. Iron deficiency anemia
D. Hemophilia

204. Glanzmann syndrome is due to : PGI 1995

A. RBC fragility disturbance
B. Neutropenia
C. Platelet dysfunction
D. Pancytopenia

205. Tissue paper normoblasts help in diagnosis of —— anemia : WB 1996

A. Iron deficiency
B. Sideroblastic
C. Aplastic
D. Hemolytic

206. A young soldier runs a cross-country race and falls down. On examination, blood is pink and urine is red. Diagnosis is : AMC 1994, 95

A. Hemoglobinuria
B. Hemosiderinuria
C. Hematuria
D. Any of the above

207. Beta thalassemia is diagnosed by : PGI 1996

A. Hb electrophoresis
B. Shultzen test
C. Fragility test
D. All of the above

208. Beta thalassemia is diagnosed in peripheral blood smear by : PGI 1996

A. Target cells
B. Nucleated RBC's
C. Anisocytosis
D. Helmet cells

209. Koilonycytes are derived from : PGI 1996

A. Immature monocytes
B. Mature monocytes
C. Mature mesenchymal cells
D. Small lymphocytes

210. In multiple myeloma which of the following is not correct for diagnosis: PGI 1996

A. Plasmacytosis
B. G-spike
C. Lytic lesion
D. Normal Alk PO4

Ans. 202. C 203. C 204. C 205. A 206. B 207. A
208. A 209. B 210. B

211. NHL with intermediate grade is : AI 1999

A. Diffuse-cleaved
B. Small noncleaved
C. Lymphoblastic
D. Small lymphocytic

212. Drepanocyte is a synonym of : AIIMS 1993

A. Burr cell
B. Target cell
C. Sickle cell
D. Stomatocyte

213. 'Stress' lymphocytes are seen in Downey Type—— infectious mononucleosis : DNB 1993

A. I
B. II
C. III
D. IV

214. Echinocytes are types of :

A. RBC's
B. Lymphocytes
C. Monocytes
D. Platelets

215. Following are hypercoagulable states except : NIMHANS 1996

A. Polycythemia
B. Protein C deficiency
C. Protein deficiency
D. Antifibrinolytic therapy

216. Hemolytic anaemia of immunologic origin occurs in following except: Rajasthan 1994

A. SLE
B. Lymphoma
C. CLL
D. Plasmodium infection

217. In thalassemia major, there is : Rajasthan 1995

A. ↑MCH
B. ↑MCV
C. ↑MCV & ↑RBC
D. ↓MCV & ↓RBC

218. Disseminated intravascular coagulation is diagnosed by : Rajasthan 1996

A. Decreased Platelets
B. Decreased Prothrombin
C. Decreased factors V, VIII & X
D. All of the above

219. Bone marrow transplantation is not useful in : Rajasthan 1996

A. Thalassemia
B. Pernicious anaemia
C. Aplastic anemia
D. Leukemia

220. A single pronormoblast gives rise to about ——— mature cells : DNB 1995

A. 6
B. 12
C. 16
D. 24

221. Thrombocytosis is a recognised feature of : UPSC 1997

A. Myelofibrosis
B. Systemic lupus erythematosis
C. Azidothymidline therapy
D. Myelodysplastic syndrome

Ans. 211. A 212. C 213. B 214. A 215. A 216. D
217. D 218. D 219. B 220. C 221. A

222. Defect in haemorrhagic disease of newborn is in : AIIMS 1997

A. Platelet B. Fibrinogen
C. PT D. BT

223. Not true of PNH is : AIIMS 1997

A. Increased LAP B. Haemoglobinuria
C. Haemolytic anaemia D. Positive Hams test

224. Increased basophil count in peripheral blood may occur in : Orissa 1998

A. Chronic myeloid leukaemia
B. Urticaria pigmentosa
C. Both
D. None of the above

225. Laboratory abnormalities most helpful in establishing the presence of haemolytic anaemia : Orissa 1998

A. Low haptoglobin level
B. Low Erythropoietic level
C. Elevated serum transferrin level
D. Low serum ferritin level

226. Type of AML often associated with disseminated intravascular coagulation (DIC) : Orissa 1999; AI 2008

A. L_3 B. M_2
C. M_3 D. M_4

227. A neonate has TLC 15000; DLC——— P35 L40 E7 and metamyelocyte 15%. Find the absolute neutrophil count : AIIMS 1999

A. 5250 B. 7500
C. 2250 D. 6000

W.228. Following are true regarding anemia of chronic disease except: AIIMS 1997, 99; Kerala 1999

A. Decreased serum Fe
B. Decreased TIBC
C. Increased ferritin
D. Increased bone marrow Fe

229. Non-Palpable purpura is seen in : AIIMS 1999

A. Henoch-Schonlein purpura
B. Mixed essential cryoglobulinemia
C. Temporal artheritis
D. Drug induced vasculitis

Ans. 222. C 223. A 224. C 225. A 226. C 227. A
228. NONE 229. D

230. About a male with 10 years history of CML, true is : **AIIMS 1999**

A. Splenomegaly is prognostic significance
B. Philadelphia chromosome is always positive
C. pH chromosome is seen in RBC myeloblast megakaryocyte
D. Thrombocytopenia indicates poorest prognosis

231. Interferons are secreted by following except : **TN 1999**

A. Monocytes B. Macrophages
C. Fibroblast D. Lymphocyte

232. In β thalassemia : **TN 1999**

A. Excess β chain B. No β chain
C. No α chain D. Normal α, β chains

233. Prothrombin time detects factors : **TN 1999**

A. 8, 9, 10 B. 9, 10, 11, 12
C. 1, 2, 5, 7, 10 D. 11, 12

234. Decrease in Osmitic Fragility causes hemolysis in : **TN 1999**

A. α thalassemia B. β thalassemia
C. Sickle cell anemia D. Meth. Hemoglobinemia

235. In reticulocytes, reticulin is formed of : **Kerala 1999**

A. Condensed chromatin B. DNA
C. RNA D. Vitamin-K

236. Following are true about HSP except : **Kerala 1999**

A. Spontaneous resolution
B. Can present with crampy abdominal pain
C. Hematuria can be a symptom
D. The purpural rashes blanch on pressure

237. Benign and malignant paraproteinemia is differentiated by : **Kerala 1999**

A. Serum total protein
B. Serum immunoglobulin
C. Serum cryoglobulin
D. Monoclonal light chain in urine

238. Spherocytosis of RBC's is a common feature in : **PGI 1999**

A. G-6-P-D deficiency B. Sickle cell anemia
C. CML D. ALL

239. Donath-Landsteiner antibody is seen in : **PGI 1999**

A. PNH
B. Waldenstrom's macroglobulinemia
C. Paroxysmal cold hemoglobinuria
D. Malaria

Ans. **230. A** **231. A** **232. B** **233. C** **234. B** **235. C**
236. D **237. B** **238. A** **239. A**

240. HbA_2 concentration in thalassemia trait is : **PGI 1999**

A. <1 B. 1-2.5
C. 2.5-3.5 D. >3.5

241. Not true regarding Waldenstrom's macroglobulinemia is : **PGI 1999**

A. Lymphadenopathy is usually present
B. Blood viscosity increased
C. IgM immunoglobulin increased
D. Hypercalcemia

242. Lacunar cells are seen in which type of Hodgkin's lymphoma : **PGI 1999**

A. Lymphocyte predominance
B. Lymphocyte depletion
C. Nodular sclerosing
D. Mixed cellularity

243. Diagnostic features of Hodgkin's lymphoma are following except : **PGI 1999**

A. Sclerosing pattern B. Atypical background
C. Absent CD-30 D. RS cell

244. If both father and mother belong to AB blood group, then which one of the following blood groups will not be possible in the off spring? **UPSC 2000**

A. "A" B. "B"
C. "AB" D. "O"

245. All the following are features of sideroblastic anaemia except : **UPSC 2000**

A. Microcytosis with hypochromia
B. Increased iron stores in bone marrow
C. Responds to pyridoxine therapy
D. Responds to folic acid therapy

246. Myelopthisic anaemia is most commonly seen in: **JIPMER 2000**

A. Hodgkins lymphoma B. Multiple myeloma
C. Metastatic carcinoma D. Leukemia

247. Thrombo modulin: **JIPMER 2000**

A. Binds with prothrombin to form thrombin
B. Binds with thrombin to cause thrombosis by forming proteins-S
C. Binds with thrombin to cause anticoagulation by forming protein-C
D. Causes fibrinolysis

Ans. **240. D** **241. D** **242. C** **243. C** **244. D** **245. D**
246. D **247. C**

248. Bone marrow aspiration is essential to diagnose : TNPSC 1995

A. Iron deficiency anaemia
B. Hemolytic anaemia
C. Megaloblastic anaemia
D. Chronic myeloid leukemia

249. LAP (Leucocyte alkaline phosphate) is increased in following except: UP 1999

A. CML B. ALL
C. PNH D. Leukemoid reaction

250. Normal platelet count is found in : UP 2000

A. Wiskott-Aldrich syndrome
B. H.S. purpura
C. Immune thrombocytopenia
D. Mayer-Rokitansky-K.H. syndrome

251. Acute promyelocytic leukaemia (AML-M_3) includes which of the following subtypes ? Kerala 2000

A. Hypergranular and hypogranular type
B. Hypergranular and hypersegmented
C. Hypergranular and microgranular type
D. Hypogranular and microgranular type
E. Hypogranular and inclusion type

252. Which is the early and relatively specific sign of immunodeficiency in HIV positive males ? Kerala 2000

A. Kaposi's sarcoma
B. Hairy Leukoplakia
C. Dental caries and periodonits
D. Herpes Zoster
E. Non-Hodgkin's lymphoma

253. Microangiopathic hemolytic anemia : PGI 2000

A. TTP B. ITP
C. Senile purpura D. CML

254. In sickle cell anaemia, true is : PGI 2000

A. Autosplenectomy due to thrombosis infarction
B. Microcytosis
C. Microcardia
D. Splenomegaly

255. Hereditary spherocytosis is due to -------- deficiency : PGI 2000

A. Spectrin B. Invertin
C. Cytokeratin D. All of the above

Ans. **248. C** **249. A** **250. B** **251. C** **252. B** **253. A**
254. A **255. C**

256. What is the most common mode of inheritance of von Willibrand's disease : AIIMS 2000

A. Autosomal dominant B. Autosomal recessive
C. X-linked recessive D. Co-dominant

257. Screening for thrombophilia is indicated in : Karnataka 2000

A. Recurrent venous thrombosis
B. Venous thromboembolism at less than 45 years of age
C. Family history of thrombophilia
D. All of the above

258. Transfusion of one unit of factor-VIII concentrate will raise the level by : Karnataka 2000

A. 1% B. 2%
C. 10% D. 25%

259. Tumor associated with polycythemia vera : AI 2001

A. Sarcoma
B Cerebral haemangioma
C. Cerebelllar haemangioblastoma
D. Sturge Weber syndrome

260. Dry marrow tap and peripheral smear has drop cells, being having anemia. Diagnosis is : AI 2001

A. Leukemia
B. Lymphoma
C. Myelofibrosis
D. Polycythemia rubra vera

261. Which of the following is a post blood transfusion complication : AI 2001

A. Metabolic alkalosis B. Metabolic acidosis
C. Resp. alkalosis D. Resp. acidosis

262. True about Haemophilia-A are following except : WB 1996; AI 2001

A. PTT increased
B. Decreased PT
C. Decreased Factor-VIII
D. Soft tissue haematoma

263. In case of allogenic Bonemarrow transplantation. Evaluation of harvested marrow is done by : AI 2001

A. Colony Stimulating Factor (CSF)-GM count, CD 34 Cell Count
B. Nucleated Cell Count, molecular marker
C. B-cell count
D. Granulocyte count

Ans. **256. A** **257. D** **258. B** **259. C** **260. C** **261. B**
262. C **263. A**

264. Following are true about polycythemia vera except : DNB 2001

A. Increased LAP score
B. Increased erythropoetin level
C. Splenomegaly
D. May cause Budd Chiari syndrome

265. Increase in Alkaline phosphatase is seen in : DNB 2001

A. CML B. Leukemoid reaction
C. Eosinophilia D. Malaria

266. β macroglobulin is derived from : DNB 2001

A. B-cells B. T-cells
C. Both D. None

267. Tissue thromboplastin activates : DNB 2001

A. Factor-VII B. Factor-IV
C. Factor-VI D. None

268. Chromosomes 15, 17 translocation is seen in which leukemia : DNB 2001

A. Ac. promyelocytic B. CML
C. CLL D. None

269. Bleeding tendency start to occur below platelet count : Rohtak 2001

A. 20, 000 B. 40,000
C. 1 lakh D. 2 lakh

270. Best stain to demonstrate sideroblasts in bone marrow is : JIPMER 2002

A. Perls stain B. Halls stain
C. Fontana stain D. Weight stain

271. Deficiency of which of the following factors does not cause an abnormality of the intrinsic pathway : SGPGI 2002

A. Factor-IX B. Factor-VII
C. Factor-XI D. Factor-VIII

272. In Henoch-Schonlein purpura, which of the following is seen : AI 2002

A. Blood in stool B. Recurrent infections
C. Thrombocytopenia D. Intracranial haemorrhage

273. All the following are seen in paroxysmal noctural haemoglobinuria except : AI 2002

A. Increased leukocyte alkaline phosphatase
B. Aplastic anemia
C. Thrombosis
D. Iron deficiency anemia

Ans. **264. B** **265. B** **266. A** **267. A** **268. A** **269. A**
270. A **271. B** **272. A** **273. A**

274. In polycythemia vera, all the following are seen except : AI 2002
A. Hyperuricemia
B. Thrombosis
C. Evolution into acute leukemia
D. Spontaneous bacterial infection

275. Levels of Hb required to maintain good body growth and normal activities in beta-thalasemic patient is : Maharashtra -2000
A. 6-8 gm%
B. 8-10 gm%
C. 10-12 gm%
D. > 12 gm%

276. Pathogenesis of PNH is : Maharashtra -2000
A. Intrinsic wall defect
B. Autoimmune
C. Genetic
D. Complement against RBC wall

277. Rouleaux formation can occur after the infusion of : BHU-2002
A. Dextran 40
B. Dextran 70
C. Gelatin
D. Human albumin

278. CD-10 is seen in : BHU-2002
A. ALL
B. CLL
C. HCL
D. CML

279. The pathogenesis of hypochromic anemia in lead poisoning is due to : AIIMS 2002
A. Inhibition of enzymes involved in heme biosynthesis
B. Binding of lead to transferrin, inhibiting the transport of iron
C. Binding of lead to cell membrane of erythroid precursors
D. Binding of lead to ferritin inhibiting their breakdown into hemosiderin

280. A 55-year old male accident victim in casualty urgently needs blood. The blood bank is unable to determine his ABO group, as his red cell group and plasma group, do not match. Emergency transfusion of patient should be with : AIIMS 2002
A. RBC corresponding to his red cell group and colloids/crystalloid
B. Whole blood corresponding to his plasma group
C. O-positive RBC and colloids/crystalloid
D. AB-negative whole blood

281. Although more than 400 blood groups have been identified, the ABO blood group system remains the most important in clinical medicine because : AIIMS 2002
A. It was the first blood group system to be discovered
B. It has four different blood groups A, B, AB, O (H)
C. ABO (H) antigens are present in most body tissues and fluids
D. ABO (H) antibodies are invariably present in plasma when persons RBC lacks the corresponding antigen

---

Ans. **274. D** **275. C** **276. D** **277. B** **278. A** **279. A** **280. B** **281. D**

282. Consider the following statements :
Factor VIII (AHF) is involved in coagulation mechanism of haemostasis: **UPSC 2002**
1. Only in extrinsic pathway
2. Only in intrinsic pathway
3. In common pathway

Which of these statements is/are correct :
A. 1 only B. 2 only
C. 1 and 3 D. 2 and 3

283. A 42-year old man was referred with a 2 weeks history of fever, weakness and bleeding gum, peripheral smear showed pancytopenia. The bone marrow examination revealed 26% blasts, frequently exhibiting Auer rods, and mature myeloid cells. An occasional neutrophil with pseudo Pelger Huet anomaly was also noted : **AIIMS 2002**
A. Acid phosphatase B. Non-specific esterase
C. Myeloperoxidase D. Toluidine blue

284. All of the following are poor prognostic factors for acute myeloid leukemias, except : **AI 2003**
A. Age more than 60 yrs
B. Leucocyte count more than 1,00,000/microl
C. Secondary Leukemias
D. Presence of t(8-21)

285. Leucoerythroblastic picture may be seen in all of the following except: **AI 2003**
A. Myelofibrosis B. Metastatic carcinoma
C. Gaucher's disease D. Thalaessemia

286. All of the following statements are true about sickle cell disease except? **AI 2004**
A. Patients may require frequent blood transfusions.
B. Acute infection is the most common cause of mortality before 3 years of age.
C. There is positive correlation between concentration HbS and polymerization of HbS.
D. Patients presents early in life before 6 months of age.

287. All of the following statements about Hairy cell leukemia are true except? **AI 2004**
A. Splenomegaly is conspicuous
B. Results from an expansion of neoplastic T-lymphocytes
C. Cells are positive for Tartarate Resistant Acid Phosphatase (TRAP)
D. The cells express CD_{25} consistently

Ans. **282. B** **283. C** **284. D** **285. C** **286. D** **287. B**

288. Microspherocytes in peripheral blood smear are seen in : **Karnataka 2005**

A. Congenital Spherocytosis
B. Autoimmune Acquired Haemolytic
C. Thalasaemia
D. All of the above

289. Megaloblastic anaemia may be caused by the following except : **UPSC 2005**

A. Phenytoin B. Amoxycillin
C. Methotrexate D. Pyrimethamine

290. HCG is raised in all the following except : **AIIMS 1992**

A. Teratocarcinoma B. Choriocarcinoma
C. Seminoma D. Yolk Sac Tumour

291. The preservative used for storing blood for transfusion is : **AIIMS 1992**

A. CPD-A B. Heparin-dextrose
C. Citrate + glucose D. EDTA

292. At what stage of erythropoiesis does hemoglobin appear ? **AIIMS 1992**

A. Early normoblast
B. Intermediate normoblast
C. Reticulocyte
D. Erthroblast

293. Auto-immune hemolytic anemia is commonly seen in: **AI 1991, JIPMER 1993**

A. ALL B. AML
C. CLL D. CML

294. Which is not a feature of Chronic lymphocytic leukemia ? **JIPMER 1993**

A. Profound anemia B. Thrombocytopenia
C. Lymphadenopathy D. More common at young age

295. Following are of B-cell origin except : **JIPMER 1993**

A. Sezary syndrome B. ALL
C. Burkitt's Lymphoma D. All of the above

296. Raised level of Serum ferritin is seen in : **JIPMER 1993**

A. Leukemia B. CRF
C. Rheumatoid arthritis D. All of the above

297. Howell Jolly bodies are seen in :

A. Megaloblastic anemia B. Post splenectomy state
C. Sickle cell anemia D. All of the above

Ans. **288. D** **289. B** **290. C** **291. A** **292. B** **293. C**
294. D **295. A** **296. D** **297. D**

298. How long can blood be stored with CPD-A? **JIPMER 1993**
A. 21 days B. 28 days
C. 35 days D. 42 days

299. ESR is greatly raised in : **TN 1993**
A. Sickle cell anemia B. Multiple myeloma
C. Acute MI D. Angina

300. Eosinophilia is a feature of : **TN 1993**
A. Thalassemia B. Spherocytosis
C. Sickle cell anemia D. Coccidiomycosis

301. Hereditary spherocytosis is due to ——— deficiency : **PGI 1997**
A. Spectrin B. Invertin
C. Cytokeratin D. All of the above

302. Non-specific esterase is present in : **PGI 1997**
A. Monocytic leukemia B. Lymphocytic leukemia
C. Erythroleukemia D. All of the above

303. Blood group antigen : **Punjab 1997**
A. Found attached to Hb molecule
B. Found in plasma proteins
C. Sometimes found in saliva
D. Found in bone marrow

304. A preponderance of lymphocytes in the differential white cell count is not seen in : **Delhi 2007**
A. Infants at birth
B. Whooping cough
C. Infants at 3 months
D. Infectious mononucleosis

305. Left shifting of neutrophils is seen in : **WB 2007**
A. Adenocarcinoma small intestine
B. Liver disease
C. Pheochromocytoma
D. Insulinoma

306. D.I.C. is seen in: **AIIMS 2007**
A. Acute promyelocytic leukemia
B. Acute myelomonocytic leukemia
C. CMC
D. Autoimmune hemolytic anemia

307. Earliest transient change following tissue injury will be : **AI 2007**
A. Neutropenia B. Neutrophilia
C. Monocytosis D. Lymphocytosis

Ans. **298. C** **299. B** **300. D** **301. C** **302. A** **303. C**
304. A **305. B** **306. A** **307. B**

308. The following protein defects can cause hereditary spherocytisis except : AI 2007

A. Ankyrin
B. Palladin
C. Glycophorin-C
D. Anion transport protein

309. ALL L_3 morphology is a malignancy arising from which cell lineage : AI 2007

A. Mature B-cell
B. Precursor B-cell
C. Immature T-cell
D. Mixed B-cell & T-cell

310. Non-specific esterase is positive in all the categories of AML except : AI 2007

A. M_3
B. M_4
C. M_5
D. M_6

311. A diabetic patient is undergoing dialysis. Aspiration done around the knee joint would show : AI 2007

A. A beta-2-microglobulin
B. AA
C. AL
D. Lactoferrin

312. Marker for Granulocytic sarcoma is : AIIMS 2008

A. CD 38
B. CD 33
C. CD 117
D. CD 154

313. A leukemia patient presenting with gum hypertrophy and hepatomegaly most likely has : AIIMS 2008

A. AML M_2
B. AML M_3
C. AML M_4
D. ALL L_2

314. The most common post-transplant lymphoma cell type is : AIIMS 2008

A. B-cell
B. T-cell
C. Null-cell
D. NK-cell

315. Poor prognostic factor in AML : AI 2008

A. Inv 16
B. T (8, 21)
C. Normal karyotype
D. Monosomy 7

316. Differential diagnosis for pancytopenia with cellular bone marrow include all of the following except : AI 2008

A. Megaloblastic anemia
B. Myelodysplasia
C. Paroxysmal Nocturnal Hemoglobinuria
D. Congenital dyserythropoietic anemia

Ans. **308. C** **309. A** **310. D** **311. A** **312. B** **313. C** **314. A** **315. D** **316. C**

317. Which of the following is the most specific marker for Hodgkin's lymphoma? **AI 2008**

A. CD 15 and CD 68
B. CD 15 and CD 30
C. CD 15 and CD 45
D. CD 30 and CD 68

318. All of the following are antigen presenting cells except : **AI 2008**

A. Langerhans cells
B. Dendritic cells
C. T-cell
D. Activated B-cell

Ans. 317. B 318. D

EXPLANATIONS OF PATHOLOGICAL ASPECTS

1. Ans.— C B cell ALL

Explanation - FAB classification of ALL

Immunological type	% of cases	FAB subtype	Cytogenetic abnormality
Pre B ALL	75	L1, L2	T (9.22), t (4:11), t (1:19)
T cell ALL	20	L1, L2	14q11 or 7q34
B cell ALL	5	L3	T (8:14),t(8:22), t(2:8)

2. Ans.— D T-cells

Histochemical stains are used to differentiate the leukemia cell populations. The periodic acid-Schiff reaction is positive in approximately 50% of cases of ALL and often shows a characteristic pattern of block positivity. A positive acid phosphatase correlates with the presence of T-cell markers.

3. Ans.— D. Tartrate resistant acid phosphatase positivity is typically seen in hairy cell leukaemia :

Hairy cells in hairy cell leukaemia (HCL) are associated with an isoenzyme of alkaline phosphatase in the cytoplasm which unlike other isoenzymes is resistant to tartorate i.e. Tartrate Resistant Acid phosphatase. TRAP stain is positive in HCL and usually negative or only weakly positive in other disorders —*Wintrobe's 11th/2468, 2470, 2471*

'TRAP' is an important tool in differential diagnosis of HCI although it is not pathognomic for the condition. The test is positive in 95% of cases of HCL and usually negative or weakly positive in other disorders.

	TRAP
B-CLL small lymphocytic lymphoma	-
Lymphoplasmacytoid lymphoma	N/A
Mantle cell lymphoma	-
Follicle center cell lymphoma	-
Malt lymphoma	-
Splenic marginal zone lymphoma	+/-
Hairy cell leukemia	+
Plasmacytoma	N/A

B-CLL: B chronic lymphocytic leukemia; TRAP : Tartare resistant acid phosphate

4. Ans. — D A diffuse proliferation of medium to large lymphoid cells with high mitotic rate :

British Journal of Haematology, 125, 294-317, 2004 Blackweel Publishing Ltd; New Biologic Indicators of Prognosis in Chronic Lymphocytic Leukemia: Vol. 18, 2, April 2004; William G. Finn, M.D. MLabs Hematology Laboratory; Wintrobe's Haematology 11th/2438; Robbins 7th/673.

The patient in question is a case of Chronic lymphocytic leukemia as indicated by the characteristic clinical picture and immunophenotypic characteristics. (Typically, CLL cells express CD_5, CD_{19}, CD_{23} and show absence of CD_{79B}, CD_{22} and FMC_7)

Histopathological examination in a case of typical CLL shows diffuse effacement of lymphocyte architecture by small to medium sized lymphocytes with clumped chromatin, indistinct or absent nucleoli and scanty cytoplasm.

The round lymphocytes may give way focally top paler areas consisting of larger round cells (prolymphocytes). These paler areas are often referred to as proliferation centers and when present are pathognomic for CLL/SLL. They contain relatively large number of mitotically active cells.

Thus, a diffuse proliferation of medium to large lymphoid cells with high mitotic rate is consistent with a histopathological picture of CLL and hence is the single best answer here.

5. Ans. — D **Inv (16) is often detected in the blasts and the eosinophils:**

This is a case of ALL with hypereosinophillic syndrome. Inv (16) is associated with AML and not ALL, and therefore represents the incorrect statement amongst the option.

WHY ALL

* Blasts were negative for myeloperoxidase and non-specific esterase

Type	Myeloperoxidase	Sudan black
AML	-	-
ALL	+	+

* Presence of positive immunological markers CD_{19}, CD_{20}, CD_{22} indicate a Ball Lineage ALL

Immunological markers for B-Cell Lineage ALL: CD19, CD_{20}, CD_{22}, CD_{79a} $_c$CD22, cCD_{79a}

Why Hypereosinophillic Syndrome : Option A Explanation

* Idiopathic hypereosinophillic syndrome is a rare condition characterized by extremely high levels of peripheral blood eosinophil counts. (80% of (70 x 109) Leucocytes were eosinophils in this patient)
* Clinical picture of dry cough, dyspnea, wheezing etc. is further suggestive of HES.
* This is differentiated from eosinophillic leukaemia by the absence of eosinophilic blast cells. (Text from case report : for option A)

6. Ans. — B **A diagnosis of plasma cell leukemia....:**

'Plasma cell leukaemia' by definition is characterized by more than 20% plasma cells in the peripheral blood. The patient in question has 14% plasma blasts in peripheral blood and thus does not classify as a plasma cell leukaemia.

7. Ans. — D **Thrombin :**

'Thrombin is essential for the culmination of the coagulation cascade and converted the soluble plasma protein fibrinogen into the insoluble fibrillator protein fibrin - It is thus perhaps the most important procoagulant and is formed from factor-II or prothrombin.'

Thus, while protein-C and protein-S are natural anticoagulants thrombomodulin has indirect anticoagulant action.

8. Ans.— D **Monosomy-7 :**

'Myelodysplastic syndromes' are a group of clonal haematopoetic stem cell diseases characterized by dysplasia and ineffective hematopoesis in one or more of the major myeloid stem lines.

Trisomy 8	10-15%
20 q	3-5%
5 q	20%
Monosomy 7	10-50%

Thus monosomy 7 and 5q are the two commonest cytogenetic abnormalities. Although 5q may be commoner than monosomy 7 in some settings, overall monosomy 7 appears more common.

9. Ans.— B **Results from an expansion of Neoplastic T-lymphocytes:**

Hairy cell leukemia is a 'B' cell neoplasm and is characterized by expansion of neoplastic B-cells (not T-lymphocytes)

10. Ans.— D **Vascular endothelium is smooth and coated with glycocalyx:**

The luminal surface of the endothelium is relatively smooth and the membrane is coated by a prominent Glycocalyx. The glycocalzy is highly charged, polysaccharide is rich felt of glycoprotein anchored to the cell membrane. Because of the high charge density the glycocalyx may contribute to the non-thrombogenic properties of the surface of the intact endothelium." - Grays

11. Ans.— D **0%**

Normal percentage of HbA_2 ranges from 1.5% to 3%

12. Ans.— D **It transports iron for erythropoiesis**

Transport of iron for erythropoesis is done by transferrin and not be Lactoferin

* **It is an iron binding protein and has high affinity for iron**
* **Lactoferrin is found in :**
  a. **specific/secondary granules in neutrophils**
  b. **many exocrine secretions and exudates - milk, tears, mucus, saliva, bile etc.**
* **It apparently exerts on antimicrobial activity by with holding iron from ingested bacteria and fungi.**

13. Ans. — B Replacement of glutamate by valine in β chain of HbA.
Substitution of valine for glutamic acid at 6th position of β chain produces HbS and hence sickle cell anemia

14. Ans. — D Howell-Jolly bodies
Chronic Manifestations of splenectomy include :
1. marked variation in size and shape of erythrocytes - anisocytosis/poikilocytes
2. Howell-Jolly bodies: nuclear remnants
3. Heinz bodies: denatured haemoglobin
4. Basophillic stippling
5. Occasional nucleated erythrocyte in peripheral blood

15. Ans. — D. Factor -IX

16. Ans. — B. Factor-XII, Factor-XI, Factor-IX, Factor-VIII

17. Ans. — D. Hepatitis-A

18. Ans. — E. None of the above

19. Ans. — C. High TIBC

20. Ans. — A. Monocytes

21. Ans. — A. Rheumatoid arthritis

22. Ans. — D. Sickle cell anaemia

23. Ans. — A. Benzene
Benzene used as a solvent in chemical, plastic, rubber and pharma industries is associated with an increased incidence of AML. Smoking, exposure to petroleum products, paint, embalming fluids, ethylene oxide, herbicides, pesticides and electromagnetic fields have also been associated with increased risk of AML.

24. Ans. — B. HbF

25. Ans. — D. Factor-VII

26. Ans. — C. Myocardial infarction

27. Ans. — C. Folic acid deficiency

28. Ans. — B. 33%

29. Ans. — B. Golden yellow

30. Ans. — B. 20,000-25,000

31. Ans. — B. SLE

32. Ans. — C. 10 days

33. Ans. — A. 17-15t
The t (15; 17) of acute promyelocytic leukemia produces a retinoic acid receptor with an abnormal cell distribution that inhibits differentiation.

34. Ans. — C. Non-Hodgkin's lymphoma
35. Ans. — A. 10%
36. Ans. — B. Epsilon 2 Delta-2
37. Ans. — A. Increase of megakaryocytes in marrow
38. Ans. — C. Adherance of platelets to vascular intima
39. Ans. — B. 0.2 to 2
40. Ans. — D. Bone marrow biopsy
41. Ans. — D. Potassium oxalate
42. Ans. — C. Obstructive jaundice
43. Ans. — C. Tear drop cell
44. Ans. — C. Haemoglobinopathies
45. Ans. — D. 2.5-4 mg/litre
46. Ans. — D. Milk
47. Ans. — C. Long standing sickle cell anaemia

    With chronic splenomegaly in certain patients, there can be pan/bi/monocytopenia that is called hypersplenism. It is primary (idiopathic) or secondary (Banti's syndrome i.e. portal hypertension with congestive splenomegaly. Malignant lymphomas, Felty's syndrome, Gaucher's disease, sarcoidosis, Kala Azar, Chronic infections (TB, brucellosis), Thalassemia, CLL, myelosclerosis.

48. Ans. — B. Reticulocytosis

    Reticulocytosis occurs 3 to 4 days after appropriate treatment and reach peak at about 10 days and after 3 weaks, the hemoglobin level increases several grams. Response to iron therapy depend on degree of deficiency, level of erythropoietin response and the health of erythroid marrow.

49. Ans. — C. Folic acid
50. Ans. — A. Kala Azar
51. Ans. — A. Platelets are effective for 9-10 days
52. Ans. — A. Antibodies to Vit. B_{12}
53. Ans. — C. Hemolytic anemia

    Leukoerythroblastic change is seen in metastatic carcinoma in BM, myelofibrosis, leukemia, multiple myeloma, Hodgkin's lymphoma, Non-Hodgkin's lymphoma and histiocytic tumours, miliary TB, severe megaloblastic anemia, severe hemolysis (in young), osteopetrosis (Albers-Schonberg disease).

54. Ans. — B. Sickle cell anemia
55. Ans. — B. Easily detached

56. Ans.— B. Protein

57. Ans.— A. Toxoplasma

Tachyzoites are able to infect and replicate in all mammalian cells except RBC's. Most of the tachyzoites are eliminated by means of humoral and cell mediated immune responses of the host. Tissue cysts containing many bradyzoites develop 7-10 days after systemic tachyzoite infection.

58. Ans.— A. Lead

59. Ans.— D. Haemolytic crisis is the usual presentation

60. Ans.— C. Renal failure

61. Ans.— D. Hemolytic anemia

62. Ans.— C. Hypofibrinogenemia

63. Ans.— A. Blockage of the pulmonary artery by agglutinated cells

64. Ans.— C. Leucopenia

65. Ans.— A. Hyperacute rejection

66. Ans.— A. Platelet aggregation

67. Ans.— C. Typhoid

In typhoid there is leucopenia. Chloramphenicol used for treatment also causes leucopenia.

68. Ans.— C. Increased leukocyte alkaline phosphatase

69. Ans.— E. HbS

70. Ans.— B. They cannot leave the circulation

71. Ans.— C. 1.055

72. Ans.— D. All of the above

73. Ans.— B. Lymphocyte

74. Ans.— A. Acute blood loss

75. Ans.— B. Mucormycosis

76. Ans.— A. Fresh blood should be used

77. Ans.— C. Paroxysmal nocturnal haemoglobinuria

78. Ans.— D. Trypsin

79. Ans.— B. Coronary arteries

80. Ans.— B. Nephrosis

In sickle cell anemia, renal medullary infarction, papillary necrosis, haematuria, CRF (with fixed low SG) may be seen in kidney.

81. Ans.— B. 4-5 years

82. Ans.— C. Factor-XII

83. Ans.— B. Large quantity is required for WBC count

84. Ans.— D. All of the above

85. Ans.— B. E
86. Ans.— D. Coralline thrombus
87. Ans.— B. Numerous lymphoblasts
88. Ans.— D. HbA + HbF + HbA_2
89. Ans.— A. Acute promyelocytic Leukaemia
90. Ans.— A. Numbers of foetal cells in maternal circulation
91. Ans.— B. They are homogenous, non-laminated
92. Ans.— D. All of the above
93. Ans.— C. 21 Days
94. Ans.— A. Idiopathic thrombocytopenic purpura
95. Ans.— C. G-6-P-D deficiency
96. Ans.— A. Sudan black
97. Ans.— C. Increased haptoglobulins
98. Ans.— E. All of the above
99. Ans.— D. All of the above
100. Ans.— B. Capillary fragility
101. Ans.— A. Angiogenic myeloid metaplasia
102. Ans.— D. Decreased number of megakaryocytes in the bone marrow
103. Ans.— A. Paroxysmal nocturnal hemoglobinuria

Pancytopenia may be seen in disorders infiltrating BM (Aleukemic/subleukemic leukemia), multiple myeloma, metastatic carcinoma, myelofibrosis, osteopetrosis), disorders involving spleen (hypersplenism), lymphomas, storage disorders, infections such as Kala Azar; TB, syphilis, primary splenic panhematopenia), Vitamin B_{12} or folate deficiency, SLE, PNH, Others (overwhelming infections, Brucellosis, sarcoidosis, pregnancy. Some refractory anemias, sideroblastic anemia) and aplastic anemia.

104. Ans.— C. Increase osmotic fragility
105. Ans.— A. Willebrand's disease
106. Ans.— C. Stool for occult blood
107. Ans.— C. Macroglobulinemia
108. Ans.— C. Detect "incomplete" antibody in the serum
109. Ans.— A. It is diagnosed by poor clot retraction
110. Ans.— A. 70% circulating and 30% in splenic pool
111. Ans.— D. Mycosis fungoides
112. Ans.— D. Idiopathic thrombocytopenic purpura

113. Ans.— D. Local stasis

114. Ans. — B. B-cell

115. Ans. — D. None of the above

116. Ans. — B. 30 minutes

117. Ans. — A. Defective haemostasis

118. Ans. — D. Widespread lymph node enlargement may occur

119. Ans. — C. Hypernephroma

120. Ans.— B. Hypothyroidism

121. Ans. — B. Decrease Immunoglobulins

122. Ans. — C. SLE

123. Ans. — C. NCE positive

124. Ans. — D. Trichinella

125. Ans. — D. Hypoproteinemia

126. Ans. — A. Balanced translocation

Cytogenetic hallmark of CML found in 90-95% of cases is t (9:22) (q34; q11). Philadelphia chromosome arises from the reciprocal 9 : 22 translocation.

127. Ans.— A. Liver

128. Ans. — A. CML

129. Ans. — C. Cryoprecipitate

130. Ans. — A. t 15 : 17

131. Ans. — D. ESR

132. Ans. — B. Newborn

133. Ans. — E. ESR

134. Ans.— C. 4-5 years

135. Ans. — A. IgG

The classic triad of myeloma is marrow plamacytosis (>10%), lytic bone lesions and a serum, and/or urine M component. IL-6 may also play a role. M-component is IgG in 53%, IgA in 25% and IgD in 1% and 20% have only light chains in serum and urine.

136. Ans. — C. Monocytes

137. Ans. — B. Type-II

138. Ans. — B. 2

139. Ans. — D. IgG

140. Ans. — B. VIII

141. Ans.— E. Malaria

In sickle cell anemia, Str. pneumoniae, H. influenzae and Salmonella infections are common.

142. Ans. — C. 1 to 5 minutes

143. Ans. — C. Hb A_2 estimation

144. Ans. — D. Splenomagly

145. Ans. — C. Not seen in orientalis

146 Ans. — A. IgG kappa light chain

147. Ans. — D. Nodular sclerosing type

148. Ans. — D. Undifferentiated type

149. Ans. — B. CML

150. Ans. — C. von Willebrand's disease
In von Willebrand's disease, BT and APTT are prolonged whereas vWf, Restocetin cofactor activity are low or normal.

151. Ans. — C. Thalassemia

152. Ans. — A. 1st week

153. Ans. — C. Low and High

154. Ans. — A. Thalassemia major

155. Ans. — D. Anaemia of chronic renal failure

156. Ans. — A. Plasmacytosis>2% on bone marrow

157. Ans. — C. Fragility of cells is increased

158. Ans. — A. 2

159. Ans. — B. APTT is normal

160. Ans. — A. Serum β2-microglobulins

161. Ans. — C. Pernicious anemia

162. Ans. — D. Miliary tuberculosis

163. Ans. — C. HbCC

164. Ans. — B. Tay Sach disease

165. Ans. — D. Chronic blood loss

166. Ans. — D. None of the above
Dohle bodies are cytoplasmic inclusions can be seen during infection and probably represent fragments of ribosome rich endoplasmic reticulum.

167. Ans. — A. HbH

168. Ans. — D. Helmet cells

169. Ans. — D. ACTH intake

170. Ans. — C. Factor-VII

171. Ans. — C. Infectious mononucleosis

172. Ans. — C. Infectious mononucleosis

173. Ans. — B. Spleen and liver resume haemopoiesis

174. Ans. — B. Serum ferritin concentration
175. Ans. — C. Thalassemic haemosiderosis
176. Ans. — D. Haemophilia
177. Ans. — C. Hemophilia
178. Ans. — B. Increased neutrophil segmentation
The finding of significant macrocytosis (MCV>100 fL) suggest the presence of megaloblastic anemia.
179. Ans. — A. Peripheral blood smear
180. Ans. — B. Capillaries
181. Ans. — C. Congestive heart failure
182. Ans. — B. F
183. Ans. — C. Beta Thalassemia major
184. Ans. — D. Idiopathic thrombocytopenic purpura
185. Ans. — C. 3 :1
186. Ans. — D. All of the above
187. Ans. — C. 280 million
188. Ans. — C. 95
189. Ans. — A. Chronic liver disease
190. Ans. — C. Calcification of islets
191. Ans. — B. B. cell
192. Ans. — B. B-Lymphocyte
193. Ans. — D. Thalassemia
194. Ans. — D. Normocytic, normochromic
195. Ans. — B. Sideroblastic anaemia
196. Ans. — B. Hypothalamus
197. Ans. — A. Platelet aggregator
von Willebrand factor is a heterogenous multimeric plasma glycoprotein with two major functions. It facilitates platelet adhesion and also acts as plasma carrier for factor-VIII. Normal plasma level is 10 mg/L.
198. Ans. — A. Extrinsic pathway of coagulation
199. Ans. — D. Pernicious anaemia
200. Ans. — D. None of the above
201. Ans. — C. Trisodium citrate
202. Ans. — C. HbS
203. Ans. — C. Iron deficiency anemia
204. Ans. — C. Platelet dysfunction

205. Ans. — A. Iron deficiency

206. Ans. — B. Hemosiderinuria

207. Ans. — A. Hb electrophoresis

208. Ans. — A. Target cells

209. Ans. — B. Mature monocytes

210. Ans. — B. G-spike

211. Ans. — A. Diffuse-cleaved

212. Ans. — C. Sickle cell

213. Ans. — B. II

214. Ans. — A. RBC's

Echinocytes (sea-urchin cell, crenated cell, burr cell) has 10-30 spicules evenly distributed over surface of RBC. There are seen in uremia, neonates, pyruvatekinase deficiency and phosphoglycerate kinase deficiency.

215. Ans. — A. Polycythemia

216. Ans. — D. Plasmodium infection

217. Ans. — D. ↓MCV & ↓RBC

218. Ans. — D. All of the above

219. Ans. — B. Pernicious anaemia

220. Ans. — C. 16

221. Ans. — A. Myelofibrosis

222. Ans. — C. PT

223. Ans. — A. Increased LAP

224. Ans. — C. Both

225. Ans. — A. Low haptoglobin level

Normal plasma levels of Haptoglobulin (Hp) is 1-1.5 gm/L. Levels are assessed by rapid latex agglutination test. Levels are reduced in intra/extracellular hemolysis, hepatocellular disease and hereditory disorders. Increased levels occur in some acute and chronic liver disease.

226. Ans. — C. M3

227. Ans. — A. 5250

228. Ans. — NONE

229. Ans. — D. Drug induced vasculitis

230. Ans. — A. Splenomegaly is prognostic significance

231. Ans. — A. Monocytes

232. Ans. — B. No β chain

233. Ans. — C. 1, 2, 5, 7, 10

234. Ans. — B. β thalassemia

235. Ans. — C. RNA

236. Ans. — D. The purpural rashes blanch on pressure

237. Ans. — B. Serum immunoglobulin

238. Ans. — A. G-6-P-D deficiency

239. Ans. — A. PNH

240. Ans. — D. >3.5

Hb Pattern in thalassemia is HbF (10-98%), HbA (very little or absent) and HbA2 (variable), usually more than 3.5% in thalassemia trait and > 2% in thalassemia major)

241. Ans. — D. Hypercalcemia

242. Ans. — C. Nodular sclerosing

243. Ans. — C. Absent CD_{30}

244. Ans. — D. "O"

245. Ans. — D. Responds to folic acid therapy

246. Ans. — D. Leukemia

247. Ans. — C. Binds with thrombin to cause anti-coagulation by forming protein C

248. Ans. — C. Megaloblastic anaemia

249. Ans. — A. CML

250. Ans. — B. H.S. purpura

251. Ans. — C. Hypergranular and microgranular type

252. Ans. — B. Hairy Leukoplakia

253. Ans. — A. TTP

254. Ans. — A. Autosplenectomy due to thrombosis infarction

255. Ans. — C. Cytokeratin

256. Ans. — A. Autosomal dominant

It is autosomal dominant with varying penetration.

257. Ans. — D. All of the above

258. Ans. — B. 2%

259. Ans. — C. Cerebelllar haemangioblastoma

260. Ans. — C. Myelofibrosis

261. Ans. — B. Metabolic acidosis

262. Ans. — C. Decreased Factor-VIII

263. Ans. — A. Colony Stimulating Factor (CSF)-GM count, CD 34 + Cell Count

264. Ans. — B. Increased erythropoetin level

265. Ans. — B. Leukemoid reaction

266. Ans. — A. B-cells

267. Ans. — A. Factor-VII

268. Ans. — A. Ac. promyelocytic

269. Ans. — A. 20, 000

270. Ans. — A. Perls stain

271. Ans. — B. Factor-VII

272. Ans. — A. Blood in stool

Skin manifestations (in 70%) and gut or joint symptoms (in 20%) are seen. Gut symptoms include colicky pain abdomen nausea, vomiting, diarrhoea,constipation, passage of blood and mucus per rectum and rarely intessuception.

273. Ans. — A. Increased leukocyte alkaline phosphatase

Patients with PNH classically present with intravascular haemolysis which is paroxysmal and nocturnal in only 25% cases. PNH results from a mutation in phosphatidylinositol glycan-A or PIGA. Leukocytic Alkaline Phosphatase is not increased.

274. Ans. — D. Spontaneous bacterial infection

PCV is a neoplasm arising in a multipotent myeloid stem cell characterized by increased proliferation and production of erythroid, granulocytic and megakaryocytic elements. About 70% patients are hypertensive and headache, dizziness and GI symptoms are common. There is increased tendency towards peptic ulceration. Symptomatic gout is seen in 5-10% patients. There is risk of bleeding. Some Patients develop AML and rarely CML.

275. Ans. — C. 10-12 gm%

276. Ans. — D. Complement against RBC wall

277. Ans. — B. Dextran 70

278. Ans. — A. ALL

279. Ans. — A. Inhibition of enzymes involved in heme biosynthesis

280. Ans. — B. Whole blood corresponding to his plasma group

281. Ans. — D. ABO(H) antibodies are unvariably present in plasma when person RBC lacks the Corresponding antigen.

282. Ans. — B. 2 only

283. Ans. — C. Myeloperoxidase

284. Ans. — D. Presence of t(8-21)
AML poor prognostic indications are : Good prognosis
* Age more than 08-21 translocation
* Lucocyte count > 20,000
* 9.22 Translocation
* 11 q 23 Translocation
* Monosomy or deletion

285. Ans.— C. Gaucher's disease
* Leucoerythroblastosis seen with myelofibrosis or myloid metaplasia etiological factors.
* Mycobacteria, fungi, HIV
* Gaucher's disease, Sarcidosis, CML, Multiple myeloma, Hairy cell Leukemia.

Degruchi clearly state that
* Gauchers & Neimann-pick diseases are the rare causes of Leucoerythroblastosis.
* MC cause is - Secondary carcinoma of bone

286. Ans. — D. Patients presents early in life before 6 months of age
287. Ans. — B. Results from an expansion of neoplastic T-lymphocytes
288. Ans. — D. All of the above
289. Ans. — B. Amoxycillin
290. Ans.— C. Seminoma
291. Ans. — A. CPD-A
292. Ans. — B. Intermediate normoblast
293. Ans. — C. CLL
294. Ans. — D. More common at young age
The median age of affection is 60 years for B-cell CLL.
295. Ans. — A. Sezary syndrome
296. Ans. — D. All of the above
297. Ans.— D. All of the above
298. Ans. — C. 35 days
299. Ans. — B. Multiple myeloma
300. Ans. — D. Coccidiomycosis
301. Ans.— C. Cytokeratin
302. Ans. — A. Monocytic leukemia
303. Ans. — C. Sometimes found in saliva

304. Ans.— A **Infants at birth**

305. Ans.— B **Liver disease**

306. Ans.— A **Acute promyelocytic leukemia**

Disseminated intravascular coagulation is associated with promyelocytic leukemia

307. Ans.— B **Neutrophilia**

Neutrophils predominate in the inflammatory infiltrate during the initial 24 hours after tissue injury (Neutrophilia).

308. Ans.— C **Glycophorin-C**

Hereditary spherocytosis is not associated with molecular abnormality in Glycophorin-C.

309. Ans.— A **Mature B-cells**

Acute Lymphoblastic Leukemias (ALL) of the L_3 (FAB) subtype are tumors of Mature B-cells (e.g. Burkitt's Lymphoma).

310. Ans.— D **M_6**

Non -specific esterase (NSE) is characteristic of M_4 (Acute Myelomonocytic) and M_5 (Acute Monocytic) Leukemia only. NSE positivity is not a characteristic feature of other subclasses of AML.

However, NSE positivity may also be seen in 15-20% of cases of M_3 or and in some cases of M_7.

NSE positivity is not a feature of M_0, M_1, M_2 and M_6 classes of AML.

311. Ans.— A **A-beta2 Microglobulin**

Patients on long term hemodialysis for renal failure develop amyloidosis due to deposition of β2 microglobulin (A β2-M). Such anyloid deposits are common in synovium, joints and tendon sheaths and hence an aspirate from the knee joint in this patient is likely to reveal β2 microglobulin.

312. Ans.— B **CD_{33}**

* Granulocytic sarcoma stains positive for both CD_{33} and CD_{117}. But CD_{33} is a better choice as explained below :
* CD_{117} Uses : Confirming diagnosis of GIST, possibly confirm chronic intestinal pseudo-obstruction.
- *Positive staining tumors with CD_{117} are :*

* AML
* Angiomyolipoma
* Angiosarcomas (50%
* Clear cell sarcoma
* CML
* Ewing sarcoma
* Epithelioid sarcoma
* Gastrointestinal autonomic tumors
* Gastrointestinal stromal tumors (GIST)
* Granulocytic Sarcoma
* Hodgkin's lymphoma (some Reed-Sternberg cells)
* Intra-abdominal fibromatosis (depends on antibody used)
* Mast cell diseases (also positive for tryptase, CD_{43}, CD_{68})
* Melanoma
* Mesenteric fibromatosis
* Metanephric adenosarcoma
* Omental mesenchymal tumor
* Osteosarcoma
* Rhabdomyosarcoma
* Sclerosing mesenteritis (variable)
* Seminomas / dysgerminomas
* Small cell lung cancer
* Synovial sarcoma (~10% usually cytoplasmic staining)
* Adenoid cystic carcinoma of salivary gland (strong staining)
* About CD_{33} :
  - Positive staining (normal) :
  * Progenitor and other myeloid cells (decreasing expression with maturation)
  - Granulocytes (low level expression)
  * Most monocytic cells
  * Mast cells
  * NK cells
  * T-cells (some)
  * Epidermal Langerhans cells (variable)
  * Circulating peripheral dendritic cells (variable)
  - Positive staining (disease) :
  * AML M0 (almost all, M_1-M_5 (75-85%), M_6, M_7 (variable), CML (90%)
  * Myeloid / Granulocytic sarcoma
  * Transient myeloproliferative disorder
  * CD_4 + CD_{56} + acute leukemias and lineage negative malignancies (weak in 44%)

* Myeloma and plasmacytoma (occasional reports)
* Aberrant expression in anaplastic large cell lymphoma
* Burkitt's lymphoma
* SLL/CLL or T-All."

313. Ans.— C AML-M_4

* "Infiltration of the gingivae, skin, soft tissues, or the meninges with leukemic blasts at diagnosis is characteristic of the monocytic subtypes (FAB M_4 and M_5).
* As FAB M_5 is not amongst the options, AML-M_4 is the single best answer.

314. Ans.— A B-cell

* "PTLDs (Post Transplant Lympho-proliferative Disorders) are almost always EBV-related, although cases unrelated to EBV have been described. The development of PTLD results from proliferation of EBV-transformed B-cell clones when patients receive immunosuppressive therapy following transplantation.

315. Ans.— D Monosomy 7

AMLs associated with t (8;21) or nv (16) have a relatively *good prognosis* with conventional chemotherapy. In contrast, the prognosis is dismal for patients with AML with prior myelodysplastic syndrome or following genotoxic therapy, possible because of damage to normal hematopoietic stem cells.

316. Ans.— C Paroxysmal nocturnal hemoglobinuria

Consistent with this view, PNH often arises in the setting of primary bone marrow failure (aplastic anemia), which can be caused by immune-mediated destruction or suppression of marrow stem cells.

317. Ans.— B CD_{15} and CD_{30}

The Reed-Sternberg cells are identified as large often bi-nucleated cells with prominent nucleoli and an unusual CD_{45}-, CD_{30}+, CD_{15}+ immunophenotype. In approximately 50% of cases, the Reed-Sternberg cells are infected by the Epstein-Barr virus.

318. Ans.— D Activated B-cell

Definition : An antigen presenting cell (APC) is a cell that presents MHC complexed foreign antigen on its surface which is recognized by T-cell receptor (TCR).

Antigen presenting cells are :

* Macrophages B. Dendritic cells
* Langerhans cells (immature dendritic cells)

CLINICAL ASPECTS

IMPORTANT TEXT FOR CLINICAL ASPECTS

CAUSES OF LACTIC ACIDOSIS

Group-A

Shock due to any cause, respiratory failure, poisoning with cyanide or carbon monoxide, profound anaemia

Group-B

Diabetes mellitus, hepatic failure, severe infection

Malignant neoplasm (lymphoma, leukaemia), fits

Drugs (biguanides, streptozocin, salicylates, isoniazid, fructose, sorbitol)

Toxins (ethanol, methanol)

Congenital enzyme defects

COMMON CAUSES OF METABOLIC ALKALOSIS

Underlying mechanism	*Clinical condition*
Loss of Na+, Cl^-, H^+ and water (ECF depletion)	Vomiting or aspiration of gastric contents Congenital chloridorrhoea* Administration of diuretics (benzothiadiazones, furosemide, bumetanide)
Potassium depletion	
Excessive mineralocorticoid activity	Primary aldosteronism, Cushing's syndrome Bartter's syndrome, adrenal enzyme defects, secondary aldosteronism Administration of liquorice, carbenoxolone
Administration of exogenous alkali	Oral or i.v. HCO_3^-, citrate Administration of gluconate, acetate, lactate.

1—A rare disorder associated with loss H^+ and Cl^- in diarrhoeal stools.

2—Alkalosis is uncommon in K^+ depletion due to primary renal disease.

3—Present in transfused blood.

CAUSES OF RESPIRATORY ALKALOSIS

- Hysterical overbreathing
- Assissted ventilation - overventilation
- Lobar pneumonia, pulmonary embolism
- Meningitis, encephalitis
- Poisoning with salicylate
- Hepatic failure

DIFFERENTIAL DIAGNOSIS OF MICROCYTIC, HYPOCHROMIC ANEMIA

	Iron-deficiency anemia	*ß-Thalassemia trait*	*Anemia of chronic disease*	*Sideroblastic anemia*
Serum iron	↓	N	↓	↑
TIBC	↑	N	↓	N
Serum ferritin	↓	N	↑	↑
Red cell protoprophyrin	↑	N	↑	↑ or N
Hb A2	↓	↑	N	↓

HEMOLYTIC ANEMIAS

Blood smear	*Additional lab tests*	*Diagnosis*
Schistocytes, helmet cells		Traumatic hemolytic anemia
	+ Coombs' test	Immunohemolytic anemia
	↑ Osmotic fragility	Hereditary spherocytosis
Spur cells	Abnormal LFT	Spur cell anemia
	+ Sucrose lysis	Paroxysmal nocturnal hemoglobinuria
Sickle cells	+ Sickle prep	Sickle cell syndromes
Target cells	Abn Hb electrophoresis	Hb C,D, etc.
Heinz bodies	Abn Hb eletrophoresis	Congenital Heinz body hemolytic anemia
	↓ G6PD	G6PD deficiency

MCQ'S FOR CLINICAL ASPECTS

1. **True about the anion gap is following except :** **AIIMS 1995**
   A. Is normally about 10-15 mmol/litre
   B. Is increased after glycol ingestion
   C. Is normal after glycol ingestion
   D. May be abnormal in myeloma
   E. May be normal with uretherosigmoidoscopy
2. **The anion gap is increased in all of the following except :** **CSE 1996; AI 1997**
   A. Ketoacidosis B. Methanol poisoning
   C. Cholera D. Chronic renal failure
3. **If Mg SO4 is given to mother, then infants develop :** **Delhi 1995**
   A. Hypocalcemia B. Hypokalemia
   C. Hyperkalemia D. Hypomagnesemia
4. **Hyperkalemia of acute renal failure may be treated by all of the following except :** **PGI 1984**
   A. Calcium chloride B. Sodium bicarbonate
   C. Hypotonic saline D. Sodium cycle resin
   E. Intravenous glucose and insulin
5. **In blood, ratio of [HCO^-] and [H_2CO_3] is :** **DNB 1989**
   A. 1 : 20 B. 20 : 1
   C. 10 : 1 D. 5 : 7
   E. 16 : 3
6. **In metabolic acidosis, respiration is :** **Delhi 1982, 83; AMC 1997**
   A. Deep and sighing B. Deep and slow
   C. Slow and superficial D. Cheyne Stokes respiration
7. **Excessive vomiting may results in :** **UPSC 1982, 87; AIIMS 1983, 88 PGI 1983, 87;AMC 1993**
   A. Hypochloremic hyponatremic alkalosis
   B. Hypochloremic acidosis
   C. Hypokalemic hypochloremic alkalosis
   D. Hyperkalemic hypochoremic acidosis

Ans. 1. C 2. C 3. A 4. C 5. B 6. A 7. A

8. **Dilutional hyponatremia is a side effect of the following except : DNB 1992**

A. Carbamazepine B. Octreotide
C. Mannitol D. Vincristine

9. **Hyercapnic acidosis has following features except : AMC 1988; AIIMS 1997**

A. Kussmaul's breathing B. Sweating
C. Collapsing pulse D. None of the above

10. **Following are complication of 1 V lipid infusion except : AIIMS 1997**

A. Lactic acidosis B. Letpsos
C. Deterioration of LFT D. Thrombocytopenia

11. **Which of the following statement is incorrect : AIIMS 1984, 85**

A. Respiratory acidosis is physiologically corrected by kidney
B. Metabolic acidosis is corrected by lungs
C. Respiration does not effectively control metabolic alkalosis
D. None of the above

12. **Primary water depletion is a recognised complication of all of the following conditions/disease states except : Manipal 1993**

A. Acute pancreatitis
B. Lithium therapy
C. Primary hyperparathyroidism
D. Toxic confusional states

13. **Hyperglycemia may be caused by following except : PGI 1998**

A. Quinine B. Encainide
C. Chlorthalidone D. Ethacrynic acid
E. Diazoxide

14. **Sodium content of one litre of isotonic saline is : PGI 1998**

A. 140 meq B. 154 meq
C. 40 meq D. 70 meq

15. **Hypovolemic shock occurs when intravascular volume is decreased by : PGI 1996**

A. 5-10% B. 15-25%
C. 30-45% D. 40-45%

16. **About hypocalcemia, true are following except : AI 1993**

A. Seen in CRF
B. Seen with primary hyperparathyroidism
C. Prolonged QTc interval
D. PTH production

Ans. **8. C** **9. A** **10. D** **11. C** **12. A** **13. A**
14. B **15. B** **16. B**

17. In Magnesium toxicity, following are true : **CMC 1998**
A. Depresses respiration B. ↑ reflex
C. ↓ HR D. Convulsions

18. Hypomagnesemia is seen in all of the following except : **AIIMS 1992, 97**
A. Chronic alcoholism
B. Chronic renal failure
C. Prolonged thiazide therapy
D. Giardiasis

19. Following are metabolic changes produced by total paraenteral nutrition except : **PGI 1986; AIIMS 1992; NIMHANS 1997**
A. Metabolic alkalosis
B. Rebound hypoglycemia
C. Hyperglycemia
D. Liver dysfunction

20. Anion gap is not increased in : **Delhi 1986, AIIMS 1992**
A. Renal tubular acidosis B. Diabetic ketoacidosis
C. Salicylate poisoning D. Starvation

21. Earliest indicator of sodium loss is : **JIPMER 1993, 98**
A. Reduced skin turgor
B. Orthostatic hypertension
C. Altered sensorium
D. Arrhythmia

22. Following Metabolic disorders are seen with total Parenteral Nutrition except :
AIIMS 1986; JIPMER 1993; AI 1994, 97; AI 1993
A. Hyperglycemia B. Hypoglycemia
C. Hyperkalemia D. Hypophosphatemia

23. In the management of hyperkalaemia all the following measures are helpful except : **PGI 1982; AI 1999**
A. Intravenous calcium B. Hypertonic dextrose
C. Insulin administration D. Haemodialysis
E. Oral administration of orange juice

24. Hyponatraemia may be related to except : **AMU 1985; AI 1999**
A. Addison's disease B. Hyperglycaemia
C. Excessive water gain D. Loss of salt
E. None of the above

Ans. 17. B 18. B 19. B 20. A 21. C 22. C
23. E 24. E

25. All the following condition except one may be associated with hypercalcinuria : **TN 1991**

A. Immobilisation
B. Metastasis in bone from carcinoma of the breast
C. Hyperparathyroidism
D. Overdosage with Vitamin-D
E. Addison's disease

26. Potassium intake is contraindicated during : **TN 1999**

A. Thiazide diuretic administration
B. Oliguric phase of acute renal failure
C. Diuretic phase of renal failure
D. None of the above

27. A patient has suffered considerable blood loss and has been oliguric for some hours. Factors that point towards acute tubular nacrosis which will not be reversed by fluid replacement include an increased in : **UPSC 1993**

A. Blood urea
B. Urinary sodium excretion
C. Urinary excretion
D. Urinary osmolarity
E. Urine volume

28. Following drugs produce hypokalemia except : **AIIMS 1986**

A. Vitamin B_{12} B. Theophylline
C. Gentamicin D. Lisonopril
E. Amphotericin-B

29. All of the following are associated with metabolic acidosis except : **Delhi 1984**

A. Acetazolamide B. Phenformin
C. Salicylates D. Spironolactone
E. Novobiocin

30. The blood picture is——pH 7.15, serum bicarbonates-10 meq/L and there is hyperventillation, diagnosis is : **UPSC 1987; ESI 1989**

A. Metabolic alkalosis B. Metabolic acidosis
C. Respiratory alkalosis D. Respiratory acidosis

31. Hypercalcemia shows following except : **BHU 1986**

A. Normal or tall T-waves
B. QRS prolongation
C. ST segment shortening
D. Shortened P-R interval
E. None of the above

Ans. **25. E** **26. B** **27. B** **28. D** **29. E** **30. C** **31. B**

W32. Which of the following are seen in hyperkalemia ? **BHU 1987**
A. P-R prolongation
B. Disappearance of P-waves
C. Increased-P wave duration
D. Decreased-P wave amplitude

33. True about Alkalosis is except : **UPSC 1992**
A. T-P phenomenon
B. Diminished T-wave amplitude
C. Depresses myocardial function
D. Sinus bradycardia

34. Hyperkalemia is suggested by : **AIIMS 1991**
A. Hyperreflexia B. Diarrhea
C. Abdominal distension D. Polyuria

35. Features potassium depletion include all of the following except : **AIIMS 1983; AP 1995**
A. Muscular weakness
B. Abdominal distension
C. Increased bowel sounds
D. Depressed tendon reflexes
E. Presence of extrasystoles

36. Respiratory alkalosis is seen in : **AI 1989**
A. Morphine poisoning B. Ethanol poisoning
C. Salicylate poisoning D. Barbiturate poisoning

37. Disequilibrium syndrome results due to : **AIIMS 1982, 84; ESI 1999**
A. Chronic renal failure
B. Haemodialysis
C. Hyperosmolar ketosis
D. Hypernatremic syndrome

38. Contraindicated in a patient with hyperkalemia: **PGI 1993**
A. Banana B. Curd
C. Cheese D. Tomato

39. The fall in calcium concentration is seen in : **Delhi 1988; Kerala 1999**
A. Respiratory acidosis B. Respiratory alkalosis
C. Metabolic alkalosis D. Metabolic acidosis

40. Least likely change in heat stroke is : **Delhi 1987**
A. Increased transminase B. Decreased calcium
C. Raised potassium D. All of the above

Ans. **32. ALL** **33. D** **34. C** **35. C** **36. C** **37. B**
38. D **39. B** **40. C**

41. Following are characterised by depletion of the intracellular water except : AIIMS 1995

A. Massive diarrhea B. Peritonitis
C. Pancreatitis D. Hepatic coma

42. Most severe alkalosis occurs in obstruction of : Manipal 1998

A. Cardiac end of stomach B. Pylorus
C. Ileocaecal region D. Colon

43. Milk-alkali syndrome consists of all of the following except : PGI 1992

A. Azotaemia B. Alkalosis
C. Hypercalcaemia D. Hypercalcuria

44. ABG analysis showed HCO_3^- >36, pH - 7.6, pO_2- 75 mm of Hg, PCO_2- 55 mmHg the probable cause would be : Kerala 1998

A. Severe pyloric stenosis for 2 hours
B. Hyperventination for 12 hours
C. HCO3 IV was given as Rx for MI
D. None of the above

45. Metabolic alkalosis may be seen in : Delhi 1984, 93

A. Low bicarbonate resorption
B. Increased potassium loss
C. Chronic renal failure
D. Diabetes mellitus

46. Which among the following statement about severe hypokalemia is true : AIIMS 1997

A. It causes neuropathy
B. It is common in severe essential hypertension
C. It diminishes deep tendon reflexes
D. It is common after persistent vomiting

47. Hypophosphatemia occurs in all of the following except : Karnataka 1994

A. Metabolic alkalosis
B. Rickets
C. Diabetes Ketoacidosis on therapy
D. Corticosteroid therapy

48. A patient is on ventilator. His pH is 7.5 with PO_2= 85 mmHg and 25 mmHg. HCO_3 = 23 mmol per litre. Most likely condition is : AI 2001

A. Resp. alkalosis B. Resp. acidosis
C. Metabolic alkalosis D. Metabolic acidosis

Ans. **41. D** **42. B** **43. D** **44. A** **45. B** **46. C**
47. D **48. A**

49. Hyponatremia with normal urinary sodium is seen in : **Delhi 1994**

A. SIADH B. Conn's syndrome
C. Cushing's syndrome D. Furesemide therapy

50. First line of treatment for a patient in shock with multiple fractures is : **AI 1994**

A. Blood transfusion B. I/V saline
C. I/V ringer lactate D. Platelets

51. Most common renal pathology in shock is : **Kerala 1994**

A. Acute tubular necrosis
B. Acute cortical necrosis
C. Renal vein thrombosis
D. Acute medullary necrosis

52. Drug of choice to treat metabolic acidosis in cardiac arrest is : **Kerala 1994**

A. Ringer lactate B. Normal saline
C. Isolyte-P D. $NaHCO_3$

53. In metabolic acidosis : **Kerala 1994**

A. HCO_3 decreased B. HCO_3 increased
C. pH increased D. PCO_2 increased

54. Hypercalcemia is not seen in : **PGI 1996**

A. Rheumatoid arthritis B. Gout
C. Polycythemia D. Leukemia

55. Metabolic causes of abdominal pain include following except : **Rajasthan 1994**

A. Uremia B. Diabetic ketoacidosis
C. C-esterase deficiency D. Sickle cell crisis

56. In hypersmolar hyperglycemic non-ketotic coma the blood glucose level is around : **C.U.P.G.E.E. 1996**

A. 55 mmol/L B. 20 mmol/L
C. 80 mmol/L D. 5 mmol/L

57. Muscular weakness due to deficiency of magnesium is enhanced by one of the following : **PGI 1997**

A. Hyperkalemia B. Metabolic alkalosis
C. Metabolic acidosis D. All of the above

58. In Hyponatremia not seen in : **AIIMS 1997**

A. Muscle twitching B. Raised ICT
C. Periodic paralysis D. Convulsions

Ans. **49. A** **50. C** **51. A** **52. D** **53. A** **54. B**
55. D **56. A** **57. B** **58. C**

59. Hypercalcemia is not seen in : **AIIMS 1997**

A. Sarcoidosis
B. Thyrotoxicosis
C. Vitamin-A intoxication
D. Phenytoin therapy

60. Calcium Gluconate is not used in CPR due to : **AIIMS 1997**

A. Hypocalcemia
B. Hypokalemia
C. Hyperkalemia
D. Calcium antagonists therapy

61. In Hypokalemia - not an ECG finding : **AIIMS 1997**

A. Sagging of the ST
B. Prominent U waves
C. Prolonged QT
D. Flattening and inversion of T

62. Consider the following statements : **UPSC 1997**
Hyponatraemia is a feature of :

1. Thiazide diuretics therapy
2. Glucocorticoid deficiency
3. Hyperaldosteronism
4. Infective diarrhoea

Of these statements

A. 1, 2 and 3 are correct B. 2 and 4 are correct
C. 1,3 and 4 are correct D. 1,2 and 4 are correct

63. Tetany may be present in all the following conditions except : **UPSC 1997**

A. Acute pancreatitis B. Hysterical hyperventilation
C. Hyperkalemia D. Hypomagnesemia

64. Not associated with hypopotassaemia is : **Orissa 1999**

A. Shortened QT interval
B. Paralytic ileus
C. Impaired concentrating ability of kidneys
D. Depressed ST segments and flattened T waves

65. A 26-year old male develops severe, acute, watery diarrhoea of 48 hours duration. He is brought to the casualty in a stuporous state. On examination, he was found to have a fast thready pulse with a systolic BP of 60 mm, Hg. The diastolic BP was not recordable. He develops sudden cardiac rhythm disturbance which settles after a few seconds. The most likely cause rhythm disturbance is : **CSE 1999**

A. Hyponatremia B. Hypocarcemia
C. Hyperkalemia D. Hypomagnesemia

Ans. 59. D 60. B 61. C 62. D 63. C 64. A
65. A

66. Hypokalemia is a deficiency of : TN 1999

A. Calcium B. Magnesium
C. Potassium D. Phosphate

67. Content of Na^+ in Ringer lactate is ——meq/L : TN 1999

A. 154 B. 121
C. 130 D. 144

68. In metabolic acidosis, treatment is: AP 1999

A. Bicarbonate B. I/V fluids
C. Ringer lactate D. K+ infusion

69. Calcium absorption occurs from : PGI 1999

A. Proximal S_1 B. Large intestine
C. Middle S_1 D. Distal S_1

70. Find the acid-base disorder in a patient on ventilator using the following blood gas value.pH 7.5; pO_2 88; pCO_2 20: AIIMS 1999

A. Respiratory acidosis B. Metabolic acidosis
C. Respiratory alkalosis D. Metabolic alkalosis

71. Treatment of Respiratory alkalosis is by : MAHE 1999

A. CO_2 inhalation B. 0.9% NaCl solution
C. O_2 inhalation D. Any of the above

72. In Parkland formula for burns, which is used? JIPMER 2000

A. Plasma B. Ringer Lartate
C. Dextran D. Blood

73. Match the following electrolyte abnormalities correctly with relevant conditions and select your answer using the codes given below : TNPSC 2000

Electrolyte abnormalities	Relevant conditions
a. Hyponatremia	1. Convulsions
b. Hypokalemia	2. Hepatic Coma
c. Hypomagnesemia	3. Cardiac arrhythmia
d. Hyperammonemia	4. Confusional state

Codes :

	a	b	c	d
A.	3	4	2	1
B.	4	3	1	2
C.	1	2	3	4
D.	4	1	3	2

Ans. 66. C 67. C 68. A 69. A 70. C 71. A 72. B 73. B

74. In a patient PO_2 in 85 mm Hg, PCO_2-50 mmHg. pH is 7.2 and HCO_3 is 20 meq/L. He is suffering from : AIIMS 2000

A. Metabolic acidosis
B. Metabolic alkalosis
C. Respiratory acidosis with compensated metabolic alkalosis
D. Respiratory acidosis with decompensated metabolic acidosis

75. A patient with pyloric stenosis secondary to peptic ulcer, complains of profuse vomiting and Na^+-125 meq/L, K^+ 2.3 meq/L and Cl^-85 meq/L, BE-8 meq/L should be given : AIIMS 2000

A. Hypertonic saline B. KCl bolous
C. Half normal saline D. Normal saline

76. Artery blood gases analysis shows O_2-85%, CO_2-20% pH 7.2 Diagnosis is : AIIMS 2000

A. Diabetic ketoacidosis
B. Respiratory alkalosis
C. Metabolic acidosis with alkalosis
D. Metabolic alkalosis

77. Aggravation of symptoms of angina in a patient when given nitrates is seen in : AIIMS 2000

A. Aortic regurgitation
B. Mitral regurgitation
C. Idiopathic hypertrophic subaortic stenosis
D. Single left coronary artery stenosis

78. Which of the following is a post blood transfusion complication : AI 2001

A. Metabolic alkalosis B. Metabolic acidosis
C. Resp. alkalosis D. Resp. acidosis

79. BMR is decreased in : Rohtak 2001

A. Myxoedema B. Cushing's disease
C. Fever D. Hyperthyroidism

80. Metabolic acidosis is not seen in : MAHE 2001

A. Cong. hypertrophic pyloric stenosis
B. Diarrhea
C. Ureterosigmoidostmy
D. Diabetes mellitus

81. How can you account for the low HCO_3^- : MAHE 2001

A. Patient hyperventilates
B. Patient hypoventilates
C. Hyperpyrexia
D. Hypothermia

Ans. 74. D 75. D 76. A 77. D 78. B 79. A 80. A 81. B

82. Hyperkalemia is seen in : **MAHE 2001**

A. Diabetes mellitus B. Hyperaldosteronism
C. Pheochromocytoma D. Myxoedema

83. In heat stroke following are seen except : **MAHE 2001**

A. Temperature is above 102 degree
B. Profuse sweating
C. Cold water compress not effective
D. None

84. Metabolic acidosis with normal anion gap is seen in : **AIIMS 2002**

A. Diabetic ketoacidosis
B. Acute renal failure
C. Diarrhoea
D. Methanol poisoning

85. A diabetic patient with blood glucose of 600 mg/dl and Na 122 meq/L was treated with insulin. After giving insulin the blood glucose decreased to 100mg/dl. What changes in blood Na level is expected : **AI 2002**

A. Increase in Na level
B. Decrease in Na level
C. No change would be expected
D. Na would return to previous level spontaneously on correction of blood glucose

86. Analysis of arterial blood gas analysis of a patient reveals pH 7.2, PO_2 54 mm Hg, PCO_2 50 mmHg and HCO_3^- below 12 mmol/lit. Most likely diagnosis is : **Delhi 2002**

A. Metabolic acidosis and respiratory alkalosis
B. Metabolic alkalosis
C. Metabolic alkalosis and respiratory acidosis
D. Metabolic acidosis and respiratory acidosis

87. The following blood profile indicate which abnormality :
pH = 7.28; HCO_3= 18 mEg/1; pCO_2 = 7 mmHg **A.P. 2002**

A. Respiratory acidosis B. Respiratory alkalosis
C. Metabolic acidosis D. Metabolic alkalosis

W.88. Hyperuricemia is seen in : **BHU-2002**

A. Nephritic syndrome B. Ecclampsia
C. Chronic renal failure D. Leukemia

Ans. **82. A** **83. B** **84. C** **85. D** **86. D** **87. C**
88. ALL

89. **All of the following cause high anion gap metabolic acidosis except :** **AIIMS 2002**

A. Lactic acidosis
B. Salicylate poisoning
C. Ethylene glycol poisoning
D. Ureterosigmoidostomy

90. **Hypocalcemia is characterised by all of the following features except :** **AI 2003; AIIMS 2003**

A. Numbness and tingling of circumoral region
B. Hyperactive tendon reflexes
C. Shortening of Q-T interval in ECG
D. Carpopedal spasm

91. **All of the following statements are correct about potassium balance, except :** **AI 2003**

A. Most of potassium is intracellular
B. Three quarter of the total body potassium is found in the skeletal muscle
C. Intracellular potassium is released into extracellular space in response to severe injury
D. Acidosis leads to movement of potassium from extracellular to intracellular fluid compartment

92. **Normal anion gap metabolic acidosis is caused by :** **AI 2003**

A. Cholera
B. Starvation
C. Ethylene glycol poisoning
D. Lactic acidosis

93. **Causes of metabolic alkalosis include all the following except :** **AI 2003**

A. Mineralocorticoid deficiency
B. Barter's syndrome
C. Thiazide therapy
D. Recurrent vomiting

94. **A 50 Kg man with severe metabolic acidosis has the following parameters: pH 7.05, pCO_2 12 mm Hg, pO_2 108 mm Hg, HCO_3 5 mEq/L base excess -30 m Eq/L. The approximate quantity of sodium bicarbonate that he should receive in half hour is :** **AI 2003**

A. 250 mEq B. 350 mEq
C. 500 mEq D. 700 mEq

Ans. **89. D** **90. C** **91. D** **92. A** **93. A** **94. A**

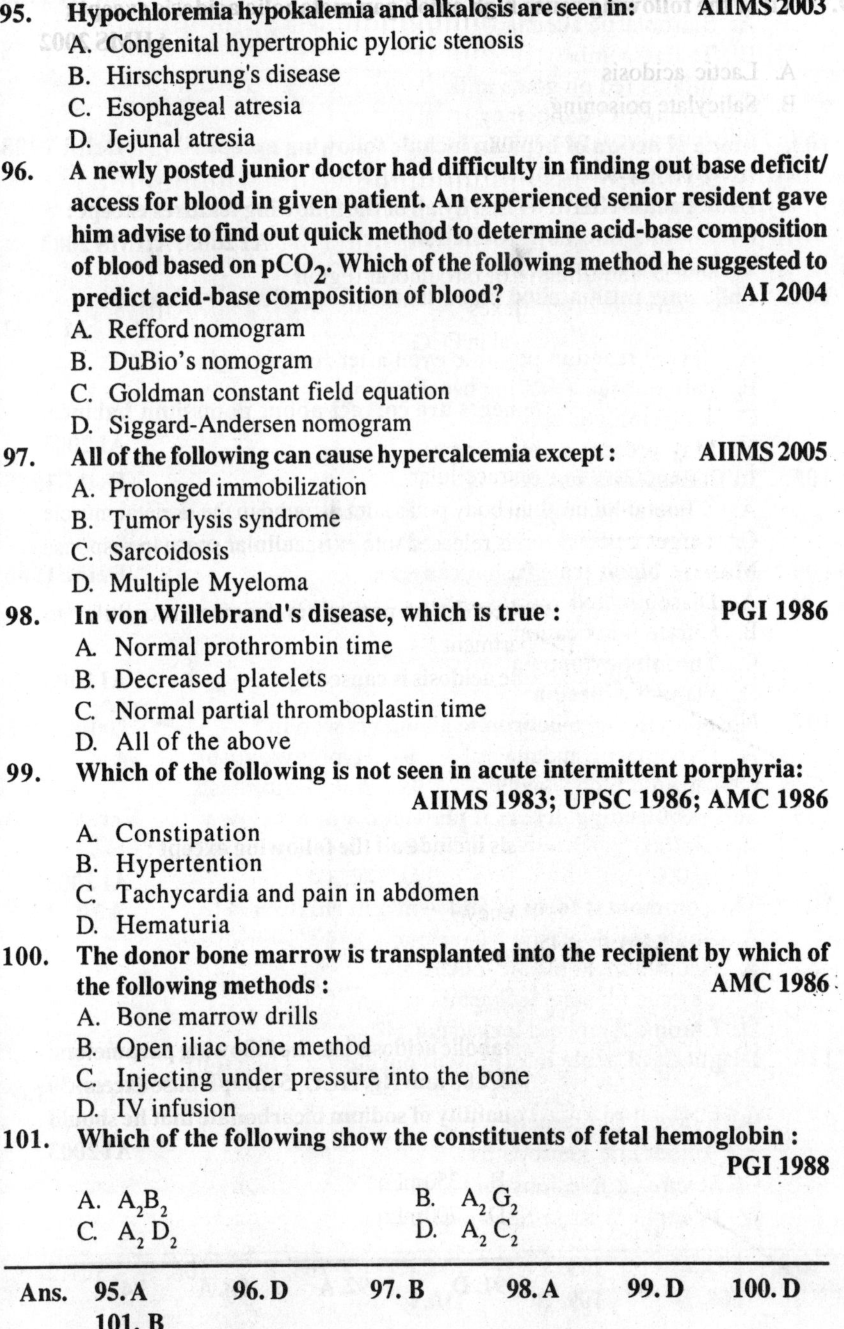

95. Hypochloremia hypokalemia and alkalosis are seen in: AIIMS 2003
A. Congenital hypertrophic pyloric stenosis
B. Hirschsprung's disease
C. Esophageal atresia
D. Jejunal atresia

96. A newly posted junior doctor had difficulty in finding out base deficit/ access for blood in given patient. An experienced senior resident gave him advise to find out quick method to determine acid-base composition of blood based on pCO_2. Which of the following method he suggested to predict acid-base composition of blood? AI 2004
A. Refford nomogram
B. DuBio's nomogram
C. Goldman constant field equation
D. Siggard-Andersen nomogram

97. All of the following can cause hypercalcemia except : AIIMS 2005
A. Prolonged immobilization
B. Tumor lysis syndrome
C. Sarcoidosis
D. Multiple Myeloma

98. In von Willebrand's disease, which is true : PGI 1986
A. Normal prothrombin time
B. Decreased platelets
C. Normal partial thromboplastin time
D. All of the above

99. Which of the following is not seen in acute intermittent porphyria: AIIMS 1983; UPSC 1986; AMC 1986
A. Constipation
B. Hypertention
C. Tachycardia and pain in abdomen
D. Hematuria

100. The donor bone marrow is transplanted into the recipient by which of the following methods : AMC 1986
A. Bone marrow drills
B. Open iliac bone method
C. Injecting under pressure into the bone
D. IV infusion

101. Which of the following show the constituents of fetal hemoglobin : PGI 1988
A. A_2B_2
B. A_2G_2
C. A_2D_2
D. A_2C_2

Ans. **95. A** **96. D** **97. B** **98. A** **99. D** **100. D** **101. B**

102. Megaloblastic anemia develops in : **PGI 1986**

A. Sidroblastic anemia
B. Thalassaemia
C. Infants fed on goats milk
D. Vitamin-C deficiency

103. Mode of action of heparin include following except : **Delhi 1988**

A. ↑ Factor-X
B. ↑ Factor-XIII
C. Inhibits thrombin formation
D. Inhibits fibrin formation

104. Following mismatched blood transfusion, all are true except : **AI 1993**

A. Severe reaction possible even after few seconds
B. Pain in back + itching usual feeling
C. ↓ Fibrinolytic activity
D. May present as bleeding

105. In thalassemia not seen is : **Delhi 1988**

A. ↑ Foetal hemoglobin
B. Reduced iron levels
C. Target cells
D. Hb A_2 normal or raised

106. Massive blood transfusion causes : **Delhi 1986**

A. Disseminated intravascular coagulation
B. Citrate intoxication
C. Thrombocytopenia
D. Platelet adhesion

107. Normocytic normochromic anemia is seen in : **Delhi 1986**

A. Hypoplastic anemia
B. Hypothyroidism
C. Chronic blood loss
D. Ankylostomiasis

108. Serious bleeding occurs if platelet count is below : **Kerala 1994**

A. 1,00,000
B. 10,000
C. 60,000
D. 40,000

109. The commonest form of leukaemia in children is : **AMC 1988**

A. Acute myeloblastic leukaemia
B. Acute lymphoblastic leukaemia
C. Chronic myeloid leukaemia
D. Chronic lymphoid leukaemia

110. Diagnosis of acute intermittent porphyria is aided by : **AMC 1988**

A. Red cell fluorescene
B. Autonomic neuropathy
C. Severe skin lesions
D. Positive Watson-Schwartz test

Ans. **102. C** **103. A** **104. C** **105. B** **106. C** **107. B** **108. D** **109. B** **110. C**

111. A 35 year old female has bleeding time 15 minutes, CT-7 minutes, PT-40 sec., PTT-30 sec., (normal-15 sec.). Correct diagnosis is : UPSC 1989

A. Hemophilia
B. Idiopathic thrombopenic purpura
C. Liver disease
D. von Willebrand's disease

112. A 40 year old male with progressive pallor with hemoglobin - 8.6 gm%, TLC-11,800/cu mm. Platelets-5,500/cu mm, Peripheral smear shows tear drops cells with anisocytosis with metamyelocytes and myelocytes. Correct diagnosis is : UPSC 1989

A. Fe-deficiency anemia
B. Megaloblastic anemia
C. Chronic myeloid leukemia
D. Leukemoid reaction

113. Neutropenia can be the feature of following except : PGI 1982

A. Acute lymphocytic leukemia
B. Typhoid fever
C. Felty's syndrome
D. Polycythemia vera

114. Myoglobinuria is seen in all the following conditions except : Delhi 1984

A. After sternous exercises
B. Crush injuries
C. Metabolic myopathies
D. Congestive cardiac failure

115. Regarding thalassaemia minor, the following is incorrect : PGI 1981

A. Hypochromic microcytic cells
B. Raised Hb A_2
C. Severe anaemia
D. Poikilocytosis and ovalocytosis

116. Poor prognosis in acute lymphatic leukaemia is indicated by all except : PGI 1982

A. Intrathoracic mass
B. Children between 2 & 10 years
C. Cranial secondaries
D. WBC around 10,000/mm^3

Ans. 111. C 112. D 113. D 114. D 115. C 116. D

117. Increased creatine kinase and alanine amino transferase are seen in : AIIMS 1984

A. Infective hepatitis B. Myopathies
C. Myocardial infarction D. Cholestasis

118. Patients homozygous for HbC may manifest following, except : AIIMS 1988

A. Marrow hyperplasia B. Intracellular crystals
C. Increased spleen size D. Increased target cells

119. Quick prothrombin time is prolonged in following, except : AMU 1988

A. Factor-V deficiency B. Factor-VII deficiency
C. Vit-K deficiency D. AHG deficiency

120. All of the following purpuras have thrombocytopenia, except : AP 1989

A. Henoch-Schonlein purpura
B. Acute leukaemia
C. Idiopathic thrombocytopenic purpura
D. Disseminated lupus erythematosus

121. When treating iron deficiency anaemia with iron, the maximal reticulocyte response occurs in the : Orissa 1991

A. 14th day B. 5th-8th day
C. 3rd week D. 4th week

122. Elevation of serum acid phosphatase is seen in : AMU 1988

A. Acute leukaemia B. Gaucher's disease
C. Multiple myeloma D. Hodgkin's disease

123. Following are associated with secondary polycythemia, except : AI 1991

A. Gastric malignancy B. Hypernephroma
C. Uterine myomata D. Cushing's syndrome

124. Red urine may be caused by following, except : AI 1991

A. Porphyrinuria B. Urobilinuria
C. Haemoglobinuria D. Myoglobinuria

125. Acute myeloblastic leukaemia is characterized by : AIIMS 1987

A. Auer rods in blast sells
B. Philadelphia chromosome
C. High leukocyte alkaline phosphatase
D. Peak incidence in childhood

126. Treatment of choice for chronic myelocytic leukaemia with high white count is : DNB 1992

A. Radiotherapy B. Busulfan
C. Leukopoiesis D. Prophylactic antibiotics

Ans. **117. C** **118. B** **119. D** **120. A** **121. B** **122. B**
123. A **124. B** **125. A** **126. B**

127. A patient with chronic myelogenous leukaemia who develops left upper quadrant pain radiating to the left shoulder probably has : UPSC 1982

A. Renal stone
B. Pancreatitis
C. Splenic infarction
D. Perforated gastric ulcer

128. A—In sickle cell anaemia, the spleen is rarely palpable :
R—Spleen undergoes autosplenectomy due to repeated infarcts: UPSC 1991

Consider the following statements :

A. Both A and R are true and R is the correct explanation of A
B. Both A and R are true but R is not the correct explanation of A
C. A is true but R is false
D. A is false but R is true

129. Haemolytic anaemias are usually associated with following, except : TN 1991

A. Increased urobilinogen
B. Erythroid hypoplasia of the marrow
C. Increased reticulocytes
D. Decreased red cell survival

130. Helmet cells and other schistocytes are suggestive of : AIIMS 1982

A. Megaloblastic anaemia
B. Iron deficiency anaemia
C. Thalassemia
D. Microangiopathic haemolytic anaemia

131. Presence of increased levels of 2,3-DPG in red cell is associated with : AIIMS 1986

A. Decreased oxygen affinity
B. Loss of red cell energy
C. Increased oxygen affinity
D. Haemolytic anaemia due to sulfa drugs.

132. Following intravenous infusion is not thrombogenic : AIIMS 1985

A. Fructulose
B. Amino acids
C. Fat emulsion
D. Alcohol

133. Thrombosthenin is : AIIMS 1986, 87

A. A coagulation factor
B. A contractile protein
C. A thrombosis promoting protein
D. A protein for stimulating platelet production

Ans. 127. C 128. A 129. B 130. D 131. A 132. B 133. B

134. Majority of chronic lymphocytic leukemia is of type : **PGI 1985, 86**

A. T-cell
B. B-cell
C. Null cell
D. Mixed B-cell and T-cell

135. In sickle cell anaemia, the pathology may be represented as : **PGI 1985; Kerala 1987**

A. HbS B Glu-Val
B. HbS A 6 Glu-Val
C. HbS B Glu-Val
D. Hbs 8 Glu-Val

136. Haemochromatosis is associated with : **AI 1990**

A. HLA A_3
B. HLA B_8
C. HLA B_7
D. HLA B_{27}

137. Philadelphia chromosome : **Manipal 1998**

A. Is a translocation from chromosome 22 to 9
B. Associated with good prognosis
C. Seen in CML
D. All of the above

138. A patient presents with a haematocrit of 20% and 300,000 platelets. The patient's blood smear reveal, relatively normal red cells. It is noted that there is no poikilocytosis, polychromasia, or basophilic stippling, and nucleated red cells are not seen in the peripheral blood. The most probable diagnosis is : **Manipal 1998**

A. Megaloblastic anaemia
B. Myelophthisic anaemia
C. Bone marrow failure
D. Iron deficiency anaemia
E. Sickle cell anaemia

139. Megaloblastic macrocytic anaemia is associated with : UPSC 1994
Consider the following statements :

1. Pernicious anaemia
2. Hypothyroidism
3. Folate deficiency
4. Hookworm's disease

A. 1, 2 and 3 are correct
B. 1 and 3 are correct
C. 2 and 4 are correct
D. 4 alone is correct

140. Match List-I with List-II and select the correct answer using the codes given below the Lists : **UPSC 1994**

List-I	List-II
I. Microcytes	(i) Pyruvate kinase deficiency
II. Macrocytes	(ii) Hypothyroidism
III. Target cells	(iii) Thalassemia
IV. Spherocytes	(iv) Splenectomy

Ans. 134. B 135. A 136. A 137. D 138. C 139. A

A. I (i), II (ii) III (iii) IV (iv)
B. I (ii), II (iii) III (iv) IV (i)
C. I (iii) II (iv) III (ii) IV (i)
D. I (iii) II (ii) III (iv) IV (i)

141. Paroxysmal nocturnal haemoglobinuria has all of the following characteristics except : UPSC 1994

A. Positive Coomb's test
B. Increased RBC osmotic fragility
C. Haemosiderinuria between attacks
D. Increased sensitivity to complement C1

142. In thrombocytopenic purpura : AMU 1987

A. Haemarthrosis are common
B. Petechia are frequently present
C. Deep dissecting haematomas are common
D. Delayed bleeding is noted frequently
E. None of the above

143. The osmotic lysis of normal red blood cells begins at a saline concentration of : UPSC 1994

A. 0.6% B. 0.48%
C. 0.36% D. 0.24%

144. Hair on end appearance in skull X-ray is characteristic of : AIIMS 1986

A. Spherocytosis B. Sickle cell anemia
C. Thalassemia D. Scurvy

145. A young female is suffering from recurrent thrombosis of big vein, abortion, thrombocytopaenia and focal-B neurological lesions. The most likely diagnosis is : UPSC 1998

A. Disseminated intravascular coagulation
B. Systemic lupus erythematosus
C. Syphilis
D. Vasculitis

146. All of the following statements are true of coagulation tests in patients with Vitamin-K deficiency except : AI 1994

A. Increased prothrombin time
B. Increased partial thromboplastin time
C. Normal thrombin clotting time
D. Decreased platelet count

Ans. 140. A 141. B 142. B 143. A 144. C 145. A
146. D

147. **PNH is due to :** **Kerala 1994**
A. Congenital membrane defect
B. Auto-immune disorder
C. Complement mediated RBC lysis
D. Acquired membrane defect

148. **Agranulocytosis is found in following, except :** **AIIMS 1983**
A. Cloxacillin B. Phenyl butazone
C. Chloramphenicol D. Hydrochlorthiazide
E. Methyl thiouracil

149. **Compounds inducing haemolysis of G-6-PD deficiency erythrocytes are :** **AMC 1984**
A. Acetanilid B. Nitrofurantoin
C. Sulphanilamide D. Primaquine
E. All of the above

150. **Tissue Eosinophilia is seen in all except :** **Delhi 1994**
A. Amoebic hepatitis B. Hodgkin's lymphoma
C. Loeffer's syndrome D. Rheumatoid arthritis

151. **Leukopenia is a common finding in :** **AP 1989**
A. Dermatomyositis
B. Periarteritis nodosa
C. Scleroderma
D. Systemic lupus erythematosus

152. **An increased serum iron and decreased iron binding capacity are found in :** **NIMHANS 1989**
A. Thalassaemia
B. Sideroblastic anaemia
C. Iron deficiency anaemia
D. Anaemia of chronic disorders
E. All of the above

153. **Normal red cell survival time is about :** **UPSC 1985; Delhi 1992**
A. 10 days B. 40 days
C. 60 days D. 120 days
E. 16 days

154. **In all of the following conditions the myeloid/erythroid ratio is decreased, except :** **TN 1990**
A. Iron deficiency anaemia B. Thalassemia
C. Sickle cell anaemia D. Cirrhosis of liver
E. In pyogenic infections

Ans. **147. D** **148. A** **149. E** **150. A** **151. D** **152. B**
153. D **154. E**

155. The following features are suggestive transformation of chronic myeloid leukemia to blast crisis except : AIIMS 1986

A. Sudden increase in splenic size
B. Onset of bleeding tendency
C. Commencement of fever
D. Appearance of lymphadenopathy

156. Polycythaemia vera is characterised by all the following features, except : TN 1991

A. Splenomegaly
B. Leucocytosis
C. Megakaryocytosis
D. Increased arterial CO_2 tension
E. Normal arterial oxygen tension

157. Sickle cell anaemia is characterized by all of the following, except: Rohtak 1985

A. Sickling of erythrocytes in vitro
B. Normocytic red cells
C. Increased osmotic fragility
D. Hyperbilirubinaemia
E. Hbs

158. The L.E. test depends on the presence of an abnormal —— with an affinity for the nuclei of cells : DNB 1989

A. Globulin B. Albumin
C. Fibrinogen D. Protein
E. None of the above

159. The E.S.R. is about 100 in : UPSC 1986

A. Pneumococcal pneumonia B. Multiple myeloma
C. Bronchiectasis D. Rheumatic fever
E. Myocardial infarction

160. G-6-P deficiency presents as : DNB 1990, Delhi 1993

A. Hemolytic anemia B. Hemoglobinuria
C. Aplastic anemia D. Hematuria

161. Not seen in multiple myeloma : AI 1993

A. Bence Jone's proteins
B. M peak in urine or serum
C. Punched out bony lesion
D. Retroperitonial lymphadenopathy

162. Petechia in scurvy is due to : AIIMS 1992

A. Platelet dysfunction B. Thrombocytopenia
C. Endothelial dysintegrity D. Clotting factor deficiency

Ans. 155. D 156. E 157. C 158. A 159. B 160. A 161. D 162. C

163. Bleeding time is prolonged in : AIIMS 1992

A. Haemophilia
B. Von Willebrand's disease
C. Henoch Schonlein purpura
D. Haemolytic telangiectasia

164. All are features of Primary Haemochromatosis except : AIIMS 1992

A. Arthritis B. Skin pigmentation
C. Diabetes D. Chorea

165. All are features of Haemolytic uremic syndrome except : AIIMS 1992

A. Segmented RBC's in peripheral smear
B. Thrombocytosis
C. Uraemia
D. Haematuria

166. Microangiopathic hemolytic anemia is a complication of all except: PGI 1993

A. Malignant hypertension B. Sickle cell anemia
C. Scleroderma D. Ecclampsia

167. Microcytic hypochromic anemia is most often due to : JIPMER 1993

A. Thalassemia B. Chronic Alcoholism
C. Hookworm infestation D. Chronic infection

168. Which of the following sites is not rich in thromboplastin : PGI 1993

A. Lungs B. Hypothalamus
C. Prostate D. Pancreas

169. Splenectomy is indicated in : AIIMS 1982, 86

A. Sickle cell anemia B. Herediatary spherocytosis
C. Hemoglobin disease D. Hodgkins lymphoma

170. A middle aged woman presents with moderate anemia with MCV of 45 toll. Which of the following will catch the diagnosis : PGI 1994

A. Serum B_{12} B. Intrinsic factor assay
C. Gastric biopsy D. Bone marrow aspiration

171. Which of the following is not true regarding hereditary spherocytosis: PGI 1994

A. Autosomal dominant inheritance
B. MCV low
C. MCHC low
D. MCH low

Ans. **163. B** **164. D** **165. B** **166. B** **167. C** **168. B**
169. B **170. A** **171. C**

172. DIC is not seen in : **AI 1995**

A. Pancreatic Ca B. Breast Ca
C. Stomach Ca D. Prostate Ca

173. Hairy cell leukaemia is characterised by following except : **PGI 1983**

A. Troublesome infections of the skin
B. Usually have considerable splenomegaly
C. Neutrophil alkaline phosphatase is very low
D. Severe neutropenia and monocytopenia is typical

174. Splenectomy as treatment is useful in following except : **PGI 1985**

A. Warm antibody haemolytic anemia
B. Hairy cell leukaemia
C. Cold antibody haemolytic anemia
D. Idiopathic thrombocytopenic purpura

175. HbA_{ic} is : **AI 1995**

A. A mutant of hemoglobin
B. Absent in 10% normal people
C. Is a result of enzymatic degradation of glucose
D. Indicates levels of glucose in blood

176. Earliest change in iron deficiency is : **AI 1995**

A. Decreased serum iron B. Decreased serum ferritin
C. Decreased TIBC D. Decreased Hb

177. When multiple myeloma presents with renal failure, which drug should not be used in combination with chemotherapy : **AIIMS 1983**

A. Melphalan B. Cyclophosphamide
C. Doxorubicin D. Carmustine

178. Deficiency of which factor is more likely to be associated with paraproteinemia involving immunoglobulin : **AIIMS 1984**

A. V B. VII
C. VIII D. XII

179. Heparin requires for its action : **PGI 1981**

A. Antithrombin-I B. Antithrombin-III
C. Antithromboplastin D. Antithrombin-VI

180. Prothrombin time evaluates the activity of following factors except : **PGI 1982**

A. II B. VII
C. IX D. X

Ans. **172. B** **173. C** **174. C** **175. D** **176. B** **177. B**
178. D **179. B** **180. C**

181. A 30-year old female presents with menorrhagia and generalised purpura for the past two weeks. There is no lymphodenopathy or sternal tenderness. Her spleen is just palpable. The Hb is 10.5%, total leucocyte count is 9.800/ cmm and the platelet count is 40,000/ cmm. There are no immature cells in the peripheral blood. The bone marrow examination is most likely to reveal : UPSC 1995

A. Megaloblastosis
B. Increased megakaryocytes with non-budding appearance
C. Hypoplastic marrow
D. Increase in myeloid/erythroid ratio

182. Following are Vit. K dependent factors except : PGI 1982

A. II B. V
C. VII D. IX

183. Life span of platelet is about : PGI 1984

A. 5 days B. 7 days
C. 10 days D. 14 days

184. Life span of granulocyte is about : PGI 1981

A. 1-2 days B. 2-3 days
C. 3-4 days D. 4-6 days

185. Leucopenia is found in following except : PGI 1981

A. Enteric fever B. Brucellosis
C. Tuberculosis D. Shigellosis

186. The total daily loss of iron amounts to about : PGI 1984

A. 0.1 mg B. 0.5 mg
C. 1 mg D. 10 mg

187. First abnormality to appear in iron deficiency anaemia is : AIIMS 1982

A. Hypochromia B. Microcytosis
C. Elliptocytosis D. Ovalocytosis

188. Ineffective erythropoiesis is a feature of : PGI 1981

A. Iron deficiency anemia
B. Sideroblastic anemia
C. Megaloblastic anemia
D. Anemia of chronic disease

189. Reticulocyte matures into an adult red cell is about : PGI 1980

A. 2 days B. 3 days
C. 4 days D. 6 days

190. $\alpha_2\delta_2$ polypeptide chain is present in : AMC 1984

A. Hemoglobin-A B. Haemoglobin-A1
C. Haemoglobin-A2 D. Haemoglobin-S

Ans. 181. B 182. B 183. C 184. C 185. D 186. C
187. B 188. C 189. A 190. C

191. One of the following drugs is used in aplastic anaemia : PGI 1980
A. Oxymethalone B. Thiazide
C. Factor-VIII D. Factor-V

192. Treatment of primary hemochromatosis is : Delhi 1982
A. Weekly venesection
B. Desferrioxamine therapy
C. EDTA therapy
D. Penicillamine

193. Peripheral blood smear in a splenectomised patient will show all the following except : DNB 1988
A. Neutrophilia B. Howell-jolly bodies
C. Target cells D. Thrombocytopenia

194. The following are the features of Thalassaemia except : AIIMS 1984
A. Bone marrow hyperplasia
B. Hair on end appearance
C. Splenomegaly is seen
D. Increased osmotic fragility

195. Blood to be stored at : UPSC 1989
A. -20°C B. +2 to +6°C
C. 0 to 1°C D. -4 to 0°C

196. Langerhan's cell histiocystosis affects : AP 1993
A. Cartilage B. Bone
C. Salivary glands D. Pancreas

197. Under normal circumstances, the predominant porphyrin in urine and faeces is : PGI 1983
A. Delta amino levulinic acid
B. Faecal protoporphyrin
C. Coproporphyrin
D. Uroporphyrin

198. In polycythemia vera, sphlenomegaly is due to : Rajasthan 1989
A. Recurrent infection B. Increased adipose tissue
C. Myeloid metaplasia D. Portal hypertension

199. Increased melanin pigmentation is a recognised feature of following except : Delhi 1982
A. Primary biliary cirrhosis
B. Chediak-Higashi syndrome
C. Haemochromatosis
D. Hyperthyroidism

Ans. 191. A 192. A 193. D 194. D 195. B 196. B
197. C 198. C 199. B

200. A 15-year old girl presents with history of 7 days' high fever, toxic appearance, anaemia, petechiae over skin ulcers in the mouth and mild hepatosplenomegaly with total count of 30,000/cumm. The most important investigation for diagnosis would be : UPSC 1998

A. Blood culture
B. Splenic puncture
C. Liver biopsy
D. Bone marrow aspiration

201. True about sickle cell anemia is all except : Delhi 1996

A. ↓ Arterial PO2
B. ↑ incidence of Gall stones
C. Isosthenuria
D. Cataract

202. In excessive intravascular haemolysis, following may be features, except : AIIMS 1982

A. Anaemia
B. Hyperbilirubinaemia
C. Splenomegaly
D. Bilirubinuria
E. Reticulocytosis

203. All of the following are features of polycythemia rubra vera, except : UP 1996

A. Increased red cell mass
B. Normal arterial oxygen suturation
C. High leukocyte alkaline phosphatase score
D. Splenomegaly

204. All of the following are true of arterial blood gas analysis except : UPSC 1998

A. Plastic syringe should be used
B. Syringe should be flushed with heparin and emptied completely
C. Syringe should be sealed with cork or a cap
D. Samples should be preserved in a cool environment

205. A 16-year old female presents with generalised weakness and palpitations. Her Hb is 7 g/dl and peripheral smear shows microcytic hypochromic anaemia; reticulocyte count = 0.8%, serum bilirubin = 1mg%. The most likely diagnosis is : UPSC 1998

A. Iron deficiency anaemia
B. Haemolytic anaemia
C. Aplastic anaemia
D. Folic and deficiency

206. Thrombotic thrombocytopenic purpura is characterised by the presence of the following features, except : UP 1996

A. Coomb's negative haemolytic anaemia
B. Normocytic normochromic blood picture
C. Renal failure
D. Neurological abnormalities

Ans. 200. D 201. D 202. D 203. B 204. D 205. B 206. B

207. Palpable purpura could occur in the following conditions, except : AI 2005

A. Thrombocytopenia
B. Small-vessel vasculitis
C. Disseminated gonococcal infection
D. Acute meningoccemia

208. The porphyrin present in normal erythrocyte haemoglobin is : AIIMS 1987

A. Coproporphyrin-I
B. Uroporphyrin-III
C. Protoporphyrin-III
D. Uroporphyrin-I
E. Coproporphyrin-III

209. A 14-years old boy was admitted with a history of pain in the right lumbar region, fever and joint pains. On examination, petechial rashes were seen on extensor surface of limbs and buttocks; urine examination showed mild albuminuria, hyaline and epithelial casts and red blood corpuscles. The most likely diagnosis is : UPSC 1996

A. Idiopathic thrombocytopoenic purpura
B. Intermittent acute porphyria
C. Henoch-Schonlein's purpura
D. Thrombotic thrombocytopoenic purpura

210. In haemochromatosis, a skin biopsy would show the presence of haemosiderin in the : Kerala 1989

A. Perifollicular area
B. Sweat glands
C. Cornified layer of skin
D. All of the above
E. None of the above

211. The serum Vitamin B_{12} level in chronic myelocytic leukaemia is : Delhi 1984

A. Normal
B. Elevated
C. Slightly decreased
D. Markedly decreased

212. Myelofibrosis is associated with : AMU 1989

A. Tuberculosis
B. Chronic myeloid leukaemia
C. Metastatic bone disease
D. Exposure to benzene
E. All of the above

213. All of the following are highly consistent with a diagnosis of myelofibrosis and myeloid metaplasia, except : Delhi 1988

A. Portal hypertension
B. Hepatosplenomegaly
C. Low leukocyte alkaline phosphatase
D. Hypermetabolic state

Ans. 207. A 208. C 209. C 210. B 211. B 212. E 213. C

214. A young person presents with a history of severe menorrhagia. She has a palpable spleen. Her bleeding time is prolonged with a normal clotting time. Platelet count is normal. The most likely diagnosis is : UPSC 1996

A. Haemophilia
B. Henoch-Schonlein purpura
C. Thrombasthenic purpura
D. Allergic purpura

215. All of the following are the causes of relative polycythemia except : UPSC 1998

A. Dehydration
B. Dengue haemorrhagic fever
C. Gaisbock syndrome
D. High altitude

216. An elderly person has been having refractory anaemia with pancytopoenia. The peripheral smear shows ring sideroblasts and 15% blast cells. The bone marrow is hypercellular. The most likely diagnosis is : UPSC 1998

A. Myelodysplastic syndrome
B. Acute myelogenous leukaemia
C. Blastic crisis of chronic myeloid leukaemia
D. Malignant infiltration of bone marrow

217. Schumm's test is done for : DNB 1988

A. B12 deficiency
B. Intravascular hemolysis
C. Phenylketonuria
D. Porphyria

218. Hoesch test is done for : AIIMS 1984

A. Porphyria
B. Vitamin-B6 deficiency
C. Vitamin-C deficiency
D. Phenylketonuria

219. In hemolytic anemia, incorrect is : PGI 1996

A. ↓ Haptoglobin
B. ↑ Urobilinogen
C. ↑ Urine bilirubin
D. ↑ Hemopexin

220. Not correct about multiple myeloma is : PGI 1996

A. Plasmocytosis
B. G-spike
C. Lytic lesion
D. Normal alkaline phosphatase

Ans. **214. C** **215. D** **216. A** **217. D** **218. A** **219. B** **220. B**

221. **Following are true of Wilson's disease except :** **Kerala 1998**
A. KF is formed just within the limbus
B. Pigment deposition between corneal endothelium and Descemets membrane
C. Pigment disappears after treatment with penicillamine
D. PenIcillamine is the drug of choice

222. **Haemoglobin is characterized by :** **DNB 1986**
A. Hydrophobic bonding in the reduced state
B. Intracellular crystallization
C. Alpha chain substitution
D. Fast migration at pH 8.6

223. **Normal serum osmolality is :** **PGI 1988**
A. 250 mosm/kg B. 270 mosm/kg
C. 280 mosm/kg D. 300 mosm/kg
E. 330 mosm/kg

224. **Following are myeloproliferative diseases except :** **Nizam 1996**
A. CLL B. CML
C. Polycythemia D. Myelofibrosis

225. **Erythropoietin may be produced in following, except :** **AMU 1986**
A. Uterine fibroids B. Colonic mucosa
C. Hepatoma D. Renal cysts

226. **Macrocytic anemia is seen in :** **AIIMS 1996**
A. Orotic aciduria B. Liver disease
C. Cu deficiency D. Uremia

227. **Iron overload is seen in all except :** **AIIMS 1996**
A. Thalassemia major B. Polycythemia vera
C. Myelophthisic anemia D. Sideroblastic anemia

228. **Basophilia is seen in :** **Orissa 1998**
A. CML B. Urticaria
C. Both D. None

229. **Intracellular inclusions in HbH disease are due to precipitated :** **Delhi 1983**
A. Delta Chains B. Gamma Chains
C. Beta Chains D. Alpha Chains

230. **In chronic lymphocytic leukaemia, lymph nodes are characterized by following, except :** **AMU 1988**
A. Firm, discrete B. Freely movable
C. Painful and tender D. Early enlargement

Ans. **221. C** **222. B** **223. C** **224. A** **225. B** **226. C**
227. C **228. A** **229. C** **230. C**

231. Basophilic stippling of RBC's on peripheral blood films is seen in : AIIMS 1984

A. Pernicious anaemia
B. Thalassemia major
C. Iron deficiency
D. Anaemia of chronic disorders

232. The diabetes of haemochromatosis is caused by : DNB 1991

A. Hepatic damage
B. Poor release of insulin
C. Sclerosis of islets of Langerhans
D. Iron deposition in pancreatic acinar cells

233. Following are true of myelofibrosis except: Kerala 1998

A. LE picture
B. Enlargement of spleen
C. Anaemia
D. ↑ WBC count

234. Commonest type of anaemia in India is : UPSC 1983, 85, 86

A. Dyshaemopoietic
B. Haemorrhagic
C. Haemolytic
D. Aplastic
E. None of the above

235. Normal blood volume in an adult male is about : AIIMS 1985

A. 50 ml/kg body wt
B. 60 ml/kg body wt
C. 69 ml/kg body wt
D. 75 ml/kg body wt
E. 79 ml/kg body wt

236. Which of the followings is not true about coagulation mechanism : AIIMS 1983, 86; ESI 86

A. Bleeding time to normal in capillary disorder
B. In disseminated intravascular coagulation. Coagulation is independent of fibrinogen
C. Bleeding time may be normal in pseudohemophilic
D. Bleeding time is increased in idiopathic purpura

237. The normal myeloid/erythroid ratio is approximately : DNB 1990

A. 1 : 4
B. 1 : 3
C. 1 : 1
D. 4 : 1
E. 2 : 1

238. Acute leukemia occurs with increased frequency in following except : PGI 1996

A. Down's syndrome
B. Bloom's syndrome
C. Klinefelter's syndrome
D. Marfan's syndrome

Ans. 231. B 232. B 233. D 234. A 235. C 236. D 237. E 238. D

239. Diamond Blackfan anaemia is ------ pure red cell aplasia : DNB 1995

A. Acute congenital B. Acute acquired
C. Chronic constitutional D. Chronic acquired

240. Exchange blood transfusion is indicated in following conditions : Rajasthan 1994

A. Infants of drug addicts mothers
B. DIC
C. Necrotizing enterocolitis
D. Hereditary fructose intolerance

241. Gum hypertrophy is seen in : AMU 1995

A. Myelogenous leukemia B. Myelomonocytic leukemia
C. Lymphocytic leukemia D. None of the above

242. A 50 year old man complains of fatigue. History is otherwise negative as is the physical examination. CBC is entirely normal. Urinanalysis is normal. The only abnormal finding is a monoclonal IgG gammopathy in the serum. Which statement is correct? UPSC 1987

A. This patient has multiple myeloma
B. Bone X-rays and a bone marrow biopsy are indicated
C. He probably has leukaemia (CML) and should be followed
D. The patient has a benign monoclonal gammopathy

243. All of the following are helpful in distinguishing myoglobinuria from haemoglobinuria, except : Rohtak 1987

A. Absorption spectrophotometry
B. Starch gel electrophoresis
C. The urine may be dark and have +ve benzidine test only in the former
D. In haemoglobinuria the serum is pink

244. Following infections are more common in multiple myeloma except : Rohtak 1992

A. Str. pneumoniae B. Staph. aureus
C. Esch. coli D. None of the above

245. Packed RBCs are prepared by : Rajasthan 1996

A. Filtration B. Centrifugation
C. Distillation D. Electrophoresis

246. Trans-retinoic acid is useful in inducing remission of : Delhi 1997

A. Acute lymphocytic leukemia
B. Chronic lymphocytic leukemia
C. Acute myelomonocytic leukemia
D. Acute myelocytic leukemia

Ans. **239. C 240. A 241. B 242. A 243. C 244. D**
245. B 246. D

247. A 16 years old male with large voluminous foul smelling stools for 4-6 days; for last 10 months he has developed anemia, most likely cause is : AIIMS 1988

A. Iron deficiency
B. Folic acid deficiency
C. Vit B_{12} deficiency
D. Pyridoxine deficiency

248. Palpable purpura is seen in following except : AMC 1987; AIIMS 1988, 90

A. ITP
B. Drug induced
C. Mixed essential cyroglobulinema
D. Vasculitis

249. Treatment of acute lymphoblastic leukaemia in child with CNS manifestations is : AIIMS 1988; UPSC 1991

A. Intrathecal methotrexate
B. Vincristine and prednisolone
C. Intrathecal vincristine
D. Intrathecal steroids and vincristine

250. Platelet aggregation is inhibited by following except : AIIMS 1982

A. Indomethacin
B. Salicylates
C. Dipyridamole
D. Phenobarbitone

251. Serum iron is raised in : AI 1989

A. Thalassemia major
B. Rheumatoid arthritis
C. Polycythemia
D. All of the above

252. False regarding FAB classification of leukemia : Kerala 1997

A. Gives prognosis
B. Classify according to lymphoblasts
C. 4 classes are present
D. None of the above

253. In a patient with leukemia in remission, Tzank smear is +ve. Next step in management would be : Kerala 1998

A. Reassurance
B. Acyclovir-IV
C. Antibiotics
D. Blood transfusion

254. Which of the following statements about patients with sickle cell disease is false ? Manipal 1992

A. Proliferative retinopathy may develop
B. Isosthenuria may occur
C. The oxyhaemoglobin dissociation curve is shifted to the left
D. A severe chest syndrome is the commonest cause of death in all age-groups.

Ans. 247. C 248. A 249. A 250 D 251. D 252. C
253. B 254. C

255. Chronic myeloid leukemia is differentiated from leukemoid reaction : AP 1997

A. Basophilic cells
B. Decreased neutrophil alkaline phosphatase
C. Increased acid phosphatase
D. Hyperuricemia

256. Which is not seen in polycythemia vera : AIIMS 1997

A. ↑ Vit. B12 binding capacity
B. ↑ Leucocytic Alk. phosphatase
C. ↑ HCL
D. Impaired ADP release to epinephrine

257. Platynchia is characteristically seen in : Rajasthan 1989

A. Copper deficiency B. Vit-B deficiency
C. Iron deficiency D. Hypomagnesemia

258. Following are used in treatment of hairy cell leukemia except : AIIMS 1997

A. Pentostatin B. Alpha 1FN
C. Steroids D. Splenectomy

259. Hemoglobinuria is not seen in : AIIMS 1997

A. CuSO4 poisoning
B. Thalassemia
C. Snake venom poisoning
D. None of the above

260. In polycythemia vera, following are true except : PGI 1997

A. Hyperuricemia B. Hypokalemia
C. Hypercalcemia D. Hyperkalemia

261. The prognosis in Hodgkin's disease is worse in all of the following situations except : Manipal 1996

A. The patient has fever on presentation
B. The patient is elderly
C. The histology is that of nodular sclerosis
D. The patient had previously been treated for the same disease

262. Consider the following statements : CSE 1996
Disseminated intravascular coagulopathy results in bleeding and is treated by :

1. Replacement of coagulation factors
2. Platelet concentrates
3. Heparin

Of these statements

A. 1,2 and 3 are correct B. 1 and 2 are correct
C. 1 and 3 are correct D. 2 and 3 are correct

Ans. **255. B** **256. C** **257. B** **258. D** **259. B** **260. B** **261. C** **262. A**

263. Pinch purpura is seen in : **Delhi 1998**
A. Secondary amyloidosis
B. Primary systemic amyloidosis
C. Pseudoxanthoma elasticum
D. Toxic shock syndrome

264. Bone marrow transplantation is indicated in all of the following except : **Orissa 1998**
A. Aplastic anemia
B. Hereditary spherocytosis
C. Thalasemia
D. AML with first remission

265. Consider the following steps : **UPSC 1997**
1. Whole blood transfusion
2. Granulocyte transfusion
3. Granulocyte monocyte colony stimulating factor
4. Antibiotics

The management of neutropaenia (WBC less than 500 cells/microlitre) would include :
A. 1,2 and 3 B. 2 and 3
C. 2,3 and 4 D. 1 and 4

266. Hand foot syndrome is due to : **PGI 1998**
A. Thalassemia B. Sickle cell anemia
C. Haemochromatosis D. Acromegaly

267. Pure red cell aplasia is produced by following except : **DNB 1993**
A. Phenytoin B. INH
C. Azathioprine D. Chlorpropamide
E. Carbamazepine

268. Leucocytosis may be produced by : **AMC 1993**
A. Lovastatin B. Nitrofurantoin
C. Corticosteroids D. Probenecid

269. Treatment of choice in idiopathic thrombocytopenic purpura is :
AIIMS 1982, 88; Delhi 1983; AMC 1984, 87
A. Steroids B. Platelet infusion
C. Splenectomy D. Androg

270. Hemolytic disease in newborn is seen if Rh factor is : **AIIMS 1987**

	Mother	**Foetus**
A.	+	—
B.	—	+
C.	+	+
D.	—	—

Ans. **263. B** **264. B** **265. C** **266. B** **267. E** **268. C** **269. A** **270. B**

271. Match List-I (Clinical condition) with List-II (Therapy) and select the correct answer using the codes given below the lists : **UPSC 1997**

List-I	List-II
A. Acute lymphatic leukaemia	1. Alpha interferon 2. deoxycorformycin, –chlorodeoxyadenosine
B. Acute myelogenous leukaemia	2. Vincristine, predinisone, 1-asparaginase
C. Chronic lymphatic leukaemia	3. Cytarabine-daunorubicin
D. Hairy cell leukaemia	4. Deoxycoformycin - 2- chlorodeoxy adenosine-fludarabine

Codes :

	A	B	C	D
A.	2	3	1	4
B.	3	2	1	4
C.	3	2	4	1
D.	2	3	4	1

272. Hemophilia with rheumatoid arthritis, analgesic of choice is : **PGI 1998**

A. Ibuprofen
B. Salicylates
C. Acetaminophen
D. Phenylbutazone

273. Hemophilia `C' is : **PGI 1984**

A. Autosomal dominant
B. Autosomal recessive
C. Sex linked recessive
D. Sex linked dominant

274. Rewarmed blood may be kept prior to use for : **PGI 1989**

A. 3 minutes
B. 30 minutes
C. 3 hours
D. All wrong

275. A 55 year old woman an anti-tuberculosis therapy developed anaemia of the microcytic hyperchromic variety not responding to iron preparations. The treatment of choice is : **PGI 1987**

A. Blood transfusion
B. Vitamin-C
C. Packed cells transfusion
D. Pyridoxine
E. Cyanocobalamine

Ans. 271. D 272. A 273. B 274. B 275. D

276. Thrombocytosis is a recognised feature of : **UPSC 1997**
A. Myelofibrosis
B. System lupus erythematosus
C. Azidothymidline therapy
D. Myeloidysplastic syndrome

277. An increase in both bleeding time and clotting time is seen in : **AIIMS 1984, 87**
A. Hemophilia
B. Christmas disease
C. von Willeband's disease
D. Idiopathic thrombocytopenic purpura

278. The erythropoiesis is decreased in following except : **AIIMS 1984**
A. Sideropenia
B. Decreased iron intake
C. Thalassemia
D. Immunosuppressive intake

279. Ferritin is seen in following except : **JIPMER 1998**
A. Liver B. Spleen
C. Bone D. Intestinal

280. AML is characterized by : **PGI 1998**
A. Philadelphia chromosome B. Auer rods
C. Hemolytic anemia D. Dohle bodies

281. Elevated serum ferritin with normal body iron stores is a feature of : **JIPMER 1998**
A. Liver damage
B. Thal. major
C. Sideroblastic anemia
D. Sickle cell anemia

282. Thrombosis is seen in following except : **AIIMS 1998**
A. Behcet syndrome B. Homocystinuria
C. Mg deficiency D. PNH

283. The decrease in hematocrit is vital if it is less than : **AIIMS 1985**
A. 40% B. 25%
C. 30% D. 20%

284. Foetal hemoglobin at birth is what percentage of total hemoglobin: **AIIMS 1985**
A. 30% B. 70%
C. 70% D. 90%

Ans. 276. C 277. C 278. C 279. B 280. C 281. A
282. C 283. D 284. C

285. In acute leukaemia, fever is because of :
UPSC 1983; AMC 1983, 87
A. Bacterial infection
B. Leukaemic infiltration
C. ↑ Metabolism of cells
D. Destruction by spleen

286. While giving blood transfusion, rigors are prevented by :
AIIMS 1982, 83; AMC 1987
A. Warming blood
B. Giving washed RBC's
C. Injection chlorpheniramine or hydrocortisone
D. All of the above

287. Best treatment of CML is : **PGI 1998**
A. Autologous BM Transplant
B. Allogenic BM transplant
C. Alpha interferon
D. Hydroxyurea

288. The commonest immunological type of multiple myeloma is :
AIIMS 1984, 85
A. IgG Kappa Light chain
B. IgA Kappa Light chain
C. IgD Lambda Light chain
D. IgM type

289. Low ESR is a feature of all of the following except : **JIPMER 1998**
A. Polycythemia rubra vera
B. Hereditary spherocytosis
C. Hereditary elliptocytosis
D. Anemia

290. Best test for assessing function of platelets is : **AIIMS 1985**
A. Bleeding
B. Clotting time
C. Clot retraction time
D. Prothrombin time

291. True about pernicious anaemia is : **AMC 1986; AIIMS 1985**
A. Totally cured by vit. B_{12} injection in a few weeks
B. Haemosiderin is decreased in bone marrow
C. Not seen in Orientalis
D. Not a cause of megaloblastic anaemia

292. Adult hemoglobin consists of chains : **AIIMS 1984, 86**
A. $2\alpha + 2\beta$
B. $2\alpha + 2\gamma$
C. $2\beta + 2\gamma$
D. $2\alpha + 2\gamma$

Ans. 285. C 286. D 287. B 288. A 289. D 290. C
291. B 292. A

293. In remission induction for AML, following are used except : PGI 1989

A. Cytarabine
B. Daunorubicin
C. Thioguanine
D. L-asparaginase

294. Daily requirement of Vitamin-K in adult is : PGI 1988

A. 20-30 microgram
B. 30-50 microgram
C. 70-140 microgram
D. More than 150 microgram

295. MC site for deep venous thrombosis is : JIPMER 1998

A. Soleal vein
B. Femoral V.
C. Popliteal V.
D. Iliac vein

296. Decreased RBC production is seen in : Manipal 1998

A. Intramuscular folate administration
B. Renal failure
C. Post gastrectomy
D. DM

297. Bone marrow transplantation as a treatment modality can be advised in all of the following cases which are newly diagnosed except : Manipal 1998

A. Combined immunodeficiency
B. CML
C. ALL
D. Aplastic anemia

298. Converging point of both pathways in coagulation is at : PGI 1988

A. Factor-VIII
B. Stuart factor-X
C. Factor-IX
D. Factor-VII
E. Factor-VIII

299. An increased red cell mass is usually seen in all of the following except: Orissa 1999

A. Polycythemia vera
B. Relative polycythemia
C. In Mansarovar area of Himalayas
D. Ayerza's syndrome

300. Ideal treatment for thalassemia is : Karnataka 1999

A. Washed cells
B. Packed cells
C. Whole blood
D. BM transplantation

Ans. **293. D** **294. C** **295. A** **296. B** **297. C** **298. B** **299. B** **300. D**

301. The following can be used to differentiate multiple myeloma from benign paraproteinemias : Kerala 1999

A. Serum protein estimation
B. Serum immunoglobulin estimation
C. Serum cryoglobulin estimation
D. Urine light chain detection

302. Which of the following is not a good screening test for hemorrhagic disease : Kerala 1999

A. Bleeding time B. Clotting time
C. Prothrombin time D. aPTT

303. Efficacy of anticoagulant heparin is best monitored by : Kerala 1999

A. PT B. aPTT
C. FDP level D. Clotting time

304. Bad prognosis in Multiple Myeloma is indicated by : PGI 1999

A. WBC>20000
B. Azotemia
C. Hypocalcemia
D. Low or normal M component production

305. True about anemia of chronic disease is : PGI 1999

A. ↓ Serum iron, ↑ serum ferritin, ↓ transferrin
B. ↑ Serum iron, ↑ serum ferritin, ↑ transferrin
C. N serum iron, N serum ferritin, N transferrin
D. ↑ Serum iron, ↓ serum ferritin, ↓ transferrin

306. A 38 year old lady on rifampicin and INH developed right femoral vein thrombosis. She was put on anticoagulant therapy but the prothrombin time remained high despite a high dose of Warfarin. Which of the following should be done: AIIMS 1999

A. Replace with acinocoumarin
B. Stop rifampicin start ethambutol
C. Low molecular weight heparin
D. Long term heparin therapy

307. A 76 year old female presented with anemia and splenomegaly. Blood examination revealed tear-drop shaped cells. Repeated bone marrow examinations were non-productive. The diagnosis: AIIMS 1999

A. Myelofibrosis B. Fe deficiency
C. CML D. All of the abovc

Ans. 301. D 302. B 303. B 304. B 305. A 306. C 307. A

308. Sachin, 25 years, complains of recurrent abdominal pain. His serum bilirubin is 2.5 and urobilinogen is positive. Hb is 8g%. Give the diagnosis: AIIMS 1999

A. Hemolytic anemia
B. G6PD deficiency
C. Urinary coproporphyrinuria
D. Protoporphyrinuria

309. A patient with eccymosis, petechiae, all the following are seen except : AIIMS 1999

A. Increased megakaryocytes in bone marrow
B. Bleeding into the joint
C. Decreased platelets in blood
D. Signs resolves by itself in 80% patients by 2-6 weeks

310. 60 year old man with perifollical haemorrhage with splinter haemorrhage, CT, PT normal, disease : AIIMS 1999

A. Vitamin-K deficiency B. Vitamin-C deficiency
C. Pyridoxine deficiency D. Vitamin-A deficiency

311. Patient with angina pectoris has intermittent pain also develops rest pain, following are given except : AIIMS 1999

A. Aspirin B. I.V. heparin
C. Bolus lignocaine D. Bolus Nitroglycerine

312. The deficiency of all of the following factors increases the incidence of thrombus formation except : UPSC 2000

A. Lipoprotein (a) B. Protein - C
C. Anti-thrombin-III D. Protein-S

313. The next two questions are based on the following case history. Study the same carefully and attempt the two questions that follow it.
A young man is admitted to the hospital with a history of bilateral cervical lymphadenopathy, progressive weight loss and fever for a few months. The investigations revealed eosinophilia and hilar lymphadenopathy.The clinical diagnosis is Hodgkin's Lymphoma. When the staging laparotomy was done, the liver, spleen and para-aortic nodes were found to be free from disease.The bone marrow biopsy was also negative.
The commonest chemotherapeutic combination to be used for this patient would consist of vincristine , prednisone, procarbazine and: UPSC 2000

A. Methotrexate B. Mitomycin-C
C. Cyclophosphamide D. Melphalan

Ans. 308. C 309. C 310. B 311. C 312. A 313. D

314. All of the following drugs are used in the treatment of CML except : MAHE 2000

A. Busulfan B. Interferon α
C. Hydroxyurea D. Melphalan

315. In congenital erythropoitic porphyria, enzyme defect is : PGI 2000

A. Uroporphyrinogen-III synthetase
B. Ferro ketolase
C. ALA synthetase
D. Proto oxidase

316. A child had Hb-6.5gm % MCV-65, MCH-15 and protoporphyria with red cell distribution width much less, is most likely to be suffering from : AIIMS 2000

A. Iron deficiency anaemia B. Thalassemia
C. Porphyria D. Megaloblastic anaemia

317. All of the following are seen in polycythemia rubra vera except : AIIMS 2000

A. Increased Vit B12 binding capacity (>900 micromols/ dL)
B. Decreased LAP score
C. Leucocytosis
D. Increased platelets

318. Blood turbulence is increased in which of the following situations : AIIMS 2000

A. Multiple myeloma B. Leukemia
C. Polycythemia D. Anemia

319. Basanti, a 25-year-old girl, presents with complaints of fever and weakness. On examination there is splenomegaly of 3 cm below the costal margin. Hb is 8 gm/dL TLC is 3,000/mm^3, platelet count is 80,000/mm^3. Which of the following is the least likely diagnosis : AIIMS 2000

A. Acute lymphocytic leukemia
B. Anemia of chronic disease
C. Aplastic anemia
D. Megaloblastic anemia

320. Lalloo, aged 54 years, who is a known diabetic patient develops cirrhosis. There is associated skin hyperpigmentation and restrictive cardiomyopathy. Which of the following is the best initial test to diagnose this case : AIIMS 2000

A. Total Iron Binding Capacity
B. Serum ferritin
C. Serum copper
D. Serum ceruloplasmin

Ans. 314. D 315. A 316. A 317. B 318. D 319. C 320. B

321. ANCA is not associated with which of the following diseases : AIIMS 2000

A. Wegener's granulamatosis
B. Henoch Schonlein purpura
C. Microscopic PAN
D. Churge Strauss syndrome

322. Most common fungal infection in febrile neutropenia : AI 2001

A. Aspergillus niger
B. Candida
C. Mucomycosis
D. Aspergillus Fumigatus

323. A patient with Hb level of 6 gm%, WBC 2000, normal, differential counting show having 6% blasts, platelets reduced to 20,000; moderate splenomegaly; diagnosis : AI 2001

A. Acute leukemia
B. Aplastic anemia
C. Lymphoma
D. ITP

324. All of the following are true regarding DIC except : AI 2001

A. Decreased platelets
B. Decreased fibrinogen
C. Decreased PTT
D. Increased PT

325. All are true regarding a hemophiliac patient undergoing dental extraction except : AIIMS 2001

A. Cryoprecipitate is required to supplement factor-VIII
B. The procedure should be done under monitored anaesthesia
C. Increased dose of lignocaine should be given for the procedure
D. Screening for HIV should be done

326. Regarding multiple myeloma, all the following statements are true except : AIIMS 2001

A. Groups of myeloma cells gives rise to plasmacytoma
B. Renal failure occurs in later stages
C. Bence Jones proteins which are excreted in urine are whole immunoglobulin molecule
D. Presents with back pain

327. A 60-year-old patient, Hashim Bhai, presented with back pain and on examination was found to have tenderness over the L_3 vertebra. His blood reports were as follows : AIIMS 2001

Hb	:	6.8 mg%
TLC	:	6500/mm3
DLC	:	$P_{55} L_{40} E_3 M_2$
ESR	:	90 mm/hr
Serum creatinine	:	3.6%
Albumin globulin ratio	:	3.9: 5.9

Ans. 321. B 322. B 323. A 324. C 325. C 326. C

The diagnosis is likely to be

A. Multiple myeloma
B. Waldenstrom's macroglobulinemia
C. Leukemia
D. Chordoma

328. In sickle cell trait, the patient does not manifest the disease because: **AIIMS 2001**

A. >50% HbS is required to cause significant dysfunction in O2 carriage.
B. The amount of HbS chain is not sufficient to form a clump and cause sicking.
C. HbA present reacts allosterically with HbS and prevents HbS from being exposed to low O2 states.
D. Inadequate HbS to form fibrin polymers.

329. Plasmapheresis is indicated for which of the following : **AIIMS 2001**

A. Wegener's granulomatosis
B. Henoch-Schonlein purpura
C. Goodpasture's syndrome
D. Acute transplant rejection

330. The cancer causing polycythenia is : **DNB 2001**

A. Mesothetioma
B. Renal cell carcinoma
C. HCC
D. Ca breast

331. Hemolytic anemia due to intrinsic red cell defect is seen in : **DNB 2001**

A. G_6PD deficiency
B. Pyruvate kinase deficiency
C. Hereditary spherocytosis
D. Autoimmune hemolytic anemia

332. In chronic Granulocyte leukemia, all are seen except : **DNB 2001**

A. Hb 12 g/dL
B. Leucocyte 50, 000/mL
C. Decreased platelets
D. Basophilia

333. Nail printing is found in : **DNB 2001**

A. Iron deficiency
B. Cirrhosis
C. Pancreatitis
D. None of the above

334. Plummer Vinson syndrome is characterised by oesophageal webs, glossitis, angular stomatitis and : **Delhi 2001**

A. Macrocytic anemia
B. Megaloblastic anemia
C. Hypochromic, microcytic anemia
D. Normochromic, normocytic anemia

Ans. 327. A 328. C 329. A 330. B 331. C 332. A 333. A 334. C

335. Prophylactic spinal irradiation is given in all except : AI 2002
A. Acute lymphatic leukemia
B. Non-Hodgkin's lymphoma
C. Hodgkin's lymphoma
D. Small cell carcinoma of lung

336. In antiphospholipid antibody syndrome all the following are seen except: AI 2002
A. Recurrent fetal loss
B. Neurological symptoms
C. Thrombocytosis
D. Prolonged APTT

337. A young lady with spontaneous abortions has a history of joint pains and fever. She currently presents with thrombosis of her leg vein. Her APTT is prolonged. The diagnosis is most likely to be : AI 2002
A. Inherited protein-C and S deficit
B. Factor-XII deficiency
C. Antiphospholipid antibody syndrome
D. Increased antithrombin-III levels.

338. In a young patient with Aplastic anemia, the treatment of choice is : AI 2002
A. ATG
B. Bone marrow transplantation
C. Danazol
D. G-CSF

339. Bone infarct is caused by : Delhi 2002
A. Sickle cell anemia
B. Myelofibrosis
C. Non-Hodgkin's lymphoma
D. Thalassemia

340. HbA_2 is raised in : Delhi 2002
A. Thalassemia
B. Sickle cell anemia
C. Myelofibrosis
D. Sideroblastic anemia

341. Which of the following is a complication of polycythemia : Delhi 2002
A. Ascites
B. Dyslexia
C. Sepsis
D. Myocarditis

342. Drug useful in mild hemophilia is : Delhi 2002
A. Corticosteroids
B. DDAVP
C. Vitamin-K
D. Tranexamic acid

343. Low leukocyte alkaline phosphatase is seen in : Delhi 2002
A. Iron deficiency anemia
B. Chronic myeloid leukaemia
C. Chronic lymphocytic leukaemia
D. Myelofibrosis

Ans. **335. C** **336. C** **337. C** **338. B** **339. A** **340. A**
341. A **342. B** **343. B**

344. Induction of remission in acute myeloid leukaemia is caused by : Delhi 2002

A. All trans-retionic acid and etoposide
B. Daunorubicin and cytarabine
C. Hydroxyurea
D. Chlorambucil and prednisolone

345. Giant splenomegaly is seen in : Delhi 2002

A. Hodgkin's disease
B. Sickle cell disease
C. Hereditary spherocytosis
D. ITP

346. A 25-year female presented with mild pallor and moderate hepatosplenomagaly. Her hemoglobin was 92 g/L and fetal hemoglobin level was 65%. She has not received any blood transfusion till date. She is most likely to be suffering from : AIIMS 2002

A. Thalassemia major
B. Thalassemia intermedia
C. Hereditary persistent fetal hemoglobin, homozygous state
D. Hemoglobin-D, homozygous state

347. The lymphocytopenia seen a few hour after administration of a large dose of prednisone to a patient with lymphocytic leukemia is due to : AIIMS 2002

A. Massive lymphocyte apoptosis
B. Bone marrow depression
C. Activation of cytotoxic cells
D. Stimulation of Natural Killer cell activity

348. Which one of the following conditions is not true regarding Myotonic dystrophy : UPSC 2002

A. Cardiac defects
B. Cataract
C. Frontal baldness
D. Enlarged testis

349. Uncontrolled action of which of the following enzymes plays a major etiological role in chronic myeloid leukemia : UPSC 2002

A. Tyrosinkinase
B. Cholinesterase
C. Galactokinase
D. Bradykinin

350. Consider the following diseases : UPSC 2002

1. Huntington's disease
2. Cystic fibrosis
3. Sickle Cell anaemia
4. Haemophilia-A

Ans. 344. B 345. C 346. C 347. A 348. D 349. A

Which of the following disorders are transmitted as autosomal recessive genetic disorders : **UPSC 2002**

A. 1,2 and 4 B. 1 and 2
C. 2 and 3 D. 3 and 4

351. One unit of fresh blood raises the Hb% concentration by : **AI 2003**

A. 0.1 gm% B. 1 gm%
C. 2 gm% D. 2.2 gm%

352. All of the following are often associated with acute intravascular hemolysis except : **AI 2003**

A. Clostridium tetani B. Bartonella bacilliformis
C. Plasmodium falciparum D. Babesia microti

353. A 63 yr old man presented with massive splenomegaly, lymphadenopathy, and a total leucocyte count of 17,000 per mm³. The flow cytometry showed CD_{19} positive, CD_5 positive, CD_{23} negative, monoclonal B-cells with bright kappa positivity comprising 80% of the peripheral blood lymphoid cells. The most likely diagnosis is : **AI 2003**

A. Mantle cell lymphoma
B. Splenic lymphoma with villous lymphocytes
C. Follicular lymphoma
D. Hairy cell leukemia

354. Memory T-cells can be identified by using the following marker : **AI 2003**

A. $CD_{45}RA$ B. $CD_{45}RB$
C. $CD_{45}RC$ D. $CD_{45}RO$

355. Which of the following is a pan-T lymphocyte marker : **AI 2003**

A. CD_2 B. CD_3
C. CD_{19} D. CD_{25}

356. A 40 yr old male had undergone splenectomy 20 yrs ago. Peripheral blood smear examination would show the presence of : **AI 2003**

A. Dohle bodies
B. Hypersegmented neutrophils
C. Spherocytes
D. Howel-jolly bodies

357. Most sensitive and specific test for diagnosis of iron deficiency is : **AI 2003**

A. Serum iron levels
B. Serum ferritin levels
C. Serum transferrin receptor population
D. Transferrin saturation

Ans. 350. C 351. B 352. B 353. A 354. D 355. A
356. D 357. B

358. Which of the following conditions is associated with Coomb's positive hemolytic anaemia: AIIMS 2003

A. Thrombotic thrombocytopenic purpura.
B. Progressive systemic sclerosis
C. Systemic lupus erythematosus.
D. Polyarteritis nodosa.

359. Which of the following marker in the blood is the most reliable indicator of recent hepatitis-B infection? AIIMS 2003

A. HBsAg
B. IgG anti - HBs
C. IgM anti - HBc
D. IgM anti - HBe

360. Elevated serum ferritin, serum iron and percent transferrin saturation are most consistent with the diagnosis of ? AI 2004

A. Iron deficiency anaemia
B. Anaemia of chronic disease
C. Hemochromatosis
D. Lead poisoning

361. Disseminated intravascular coagulation (DIC) differs from thrombotic thrombocytopenic purpura. In this reference the DIC is most likely characterized by: AI 2004

A. Significant numbers of schizocytes
B. A brisk reticulocutosis
C. Decreased coagulation factor levels
D. Significant thrombocytopenia

362. An 80 years old asymptomatic woman was detected to have a monoclonal spike on serum electrophoresis (IgG levels 1.5 g/dL). Bone marrow revealed plasma cells of 8%. The most likely diagnosis is? AI 2004

A. Multiple myeloma
B. Indolent myeloma
C. Monoclonal gammopathy of unknown significance
D. Waldenstrom's macroglobulinemia

363. Which one of the following platelet counts is usually associated with increased incidence of spontaneous bleeding ? UPSC 2004

A. Greater than 80,000/mm3
B. 40,000/mm3-50,000/mm3
C. 20,000/mm3-40,000/mm3
D. Less than 20,000/mm3

364. All of the following can cause of megakaryocyte thrombocytopenia, except : AIIMS 2004

A. Idiopathic thrombocytopenic purpura
B. Systemic lupus erythematosus
C. Aplastic anemia
D. Disseminated intravascular coagulation (DIC)

Ans. 358. C 359. C 360. C 361. C 362. C 363. D 364. C

365. The following may be abnormal in disseminated intravascular coagulation, except : AIIMS 2004

A. Prothrombin time B. Activated partial thromboplastin time

C. D-dimer levels D. Clot solubility

366. Laboratory evaluation for the differential diagnosis of chronic myeloproliferative disorders includes all of the following, except : AIIMS 2004

A. Chromosomal evaluation

B. Bone marrow aspiration

C. Flow-cytometric analysis

D. Determination of red blood cells mass

367. An 71 yrs. old patient of acute leukemia is admitted with febrile neutropenia. On day four of being treated with broad-spectrum antibiotics, his fever increases, X-ray chest shows bilateral fluffy infiltrates. Which of the following should be the most appropriate next step in the management? AIIMS 2004

A. Add antiviral therapy B. Add antifungal therapy

C. Add cotrimoxazole D. Continue chemotherapy

368. A patient is admitted with 3rd episode of deep venous thrombosis. There is no history of any associated medical illness. All of the following investigations are required for establishing the diagnosis, except : AIIMS 2004

A. Protein C deficiency . B. Antithrombin-III deficiency

C. Antibodies to factor-VIII D. Antibodies to cardiolipin

369. Which one of the following is not a criterion for making a diagnosis of chronic myeloid leukemia in accelerated phase : AIIMS 2004

A. Blasts 10-90% of WBC's in peripheral blood

B. Basophils 10-19% of WBC's in peripheral blood

C. Increasing spleen size unresponsive to therapy

D. Persistent thrombocytosis (>1000 x 109/L unresponsive to therapy).

370. CD_{19} positive, CD_{22} positive, CD_{103} positive monoclonal B-cells with bright kappa positivity were found to comprise 60% of the peripheral blood lymphoid cells on flow cytometric analysis in a 55 years old man with massive splenomegaly and a total leucocyte count of 3.3 x 109/L. Which one of the following is the most likely diagnosis is : AIIMS 2004

A. Splenic lymphoma with villous lymphocytes

B. Mantle cell lymphoma

C. B-cell prolymphocytic leukemia

D. Hairy cell leukemia

Ans. 365. D 366. C 367. B 368. C 369. B 370. D

371. The coagulation profile in a 13-years old girl with Menorrhagia having von Willebrands disease is : AI 2005

A. Isolated prolonged PTT with a normal PT
B. Isolated prolonged PT with a normal PTT
C. Prolongation of both PT and PTT
D. Prolongation of thrombin time

372. The most common leukocytoclastic vasculitis affecting children is : AI 2005

A. Takayasu disease
B. Mucocutaneous lymph node syndrome (Kawasaki disease)
C. Henoch Schonelin purpura
D. Polyartheritis nodosa

373. Diagnosis of beta Thalassemia is established by : AI 2005

A. NESTROFT Test
B. HbA1 C estimation
C. Hb electrophoresis
D. Target cells in peripheral smear.

374. Best prognosis is seen in which AML : SGPGI 2002

A. M_6 B. M_1
C. M_7 D. M_3

375. Poor prognostic indicator of ALL is : AIIMS 2002

A. Female sex
B. Age > 1 yr
C. Leucocyte count < 50,000/mm3
D. Hypoploidy

376. A child died soon after birth. On examination there was hepato-splenomegaly. The most probable diagnosis was : AIIMS 2002

A. α-thalassemia
B. Homozygous β-thalassemia
C. Hereditary spherocytosis
D. Sickle cell anemia

377. True statement about acute lymphoblastic leukemia is : Delhi 2002

A. Lymphoblasts show azurophilic granules in cytoplasm
B. Usually are of B-cell origin
C. TDt is present in 5% of ALL
D. Prognosis is good for surface Ig positive B-cell ALL.

Ans. **371. A** **372. C** **373. C** **374. D** **375. D** **376. A** **377. B**

378. In which one of the following conditions Dactylitis cannot be seen : UPSC 2002

A. Sickle-cell anemia
B. Beta thalassemia
C. Congenital syphilis
D. Tuberculosis

379. Spleen is palpable in all haemolytic anemias in a child of 8 years of age, except in : UPSC 2002

A. Thalassemia
B. Spherocytosis
C. Sickle-cell anemia
D. Haemolysis in malaria

380. A couple with a family history of beta thalassemia major in a distant relative, has come for counselling. The husband has HbA2 of 4.8% and the wife has HbA_2 of 2.3%. The risk of having a child with beta thalaessemia major is : AI 2003

A. 50%
B. 25%
C. 5%
D. 0%

381. Which of the following drugs will prevent platelet aggregation : AMC 1999

A. Paracetamol
B. Sulfonamides
C. I.N.H
D. Aspirin

382. A positive coomb's test in absence of haemolysis, may be seen with administration of : UPSC 1995

A. Cephalothin
B. Ampicillin
C. Nalidixic acid
D. Carbenicillin

383. Major indication for intrauterine transfusion of foetus is : AIIMS 1982, 92

A. Bradycardia and foetal distress
B. Sickle cell anaemia
C. Erythroblastosis foetalis
D. None of the above

384. Most common complication of intrauterine transfusion is : PGI 1983, 99

A. Graft versus host reaction
B. Premature onset of labour
C. Transfusion reaction
D. None of the above

385. Breakdown of 1 gm of haemoglobin yields about : AIIMS 1986, 90

A. 20 mg bilirubin
B. 35 mg bilirubin
C. 5 mg bilirubin
D. 1 mg bilirubin

386. Hazards of exchange transfusion include following, except : AIIMS 1993

A. Oligaemic shock
B. Citrate tetany
C. Cardiac arrest
D. Hypokalaemia

Ans. **378. B** **379. C** **380. D** **381. D** **382. A** **383. C** **384. C** **385. B** **386. D**

387. Foetal blood in the maternal circulation is detected by : AIIMS 1982, 88, 90; Delhi 1983; ESI 1994

A. Hemoglobin estimation B. Optic density
C. Spectrophotometer D. Kleihauer test

388. The least common leukaemia in a child is : UPSC 1983, 88; AIIMS 1999

A. Acute lymphocytic leukaemia
B. Acute meyloblastic leukaemia
C. Acute non-lymphocytic leukaemia
D. Chronic myeloid leukaemia

389. The word, "thalassemia" literally means : AMC 1994

A. Fatal illness B. Great curse
C. Great sea D. Punishment

390. Structural haemoglobinopathy is : Delhi 1996

A. β-Thalassemia B. α-Thalassemia
C. Hb-H disease D. Sickle cell anemia

391. Hemophilia is because of deficiency of : Delhi 1996

A. Factor-VIII B. Factor-IX
C. ↑ Bleeding time D. ↑ Prothrombin time

392. Hypertransfusion in Thalassemia is given by : Delhi 1990

A. 6 gm% B. 8 gm%
C. 10 gm% D. 12 gm%

393. Anaphylactoid purpura : AIIMS 1992

A. Is the same entity as idiopathic thrombocytopenic purpura
B. Is the same entity as Henoch-Schonlein purpura
C. Is the same entity as black measles
D. May cause acute chest pain

394. Lymphocytosis is seen in except : Rajasthan 1998

A. TB B. Typhoid
C. Brucellosis D. Infant

395. Thrombocytopenia is seen in following except : AIIMS 1998

A. Hemolytic uremic syndrome
B. Immune thrombocytopenia
C. Henoch Schonlein purpura
D. Thrombocytopenic purpura

396. A 5 year old child has anaemia of long duration. The investigation to be done is : AIIMS 1987, 98

A. Estimation of Hb% B. RBC count
C. Peripheral smear D. PVC

Ans. 387. D 388. D 389. C 390. D 391. A 392. C
393. B 394. D 395. C 396. C

397. A child with congenital haemolytic anaemia will show all these features, except : AIIMS 1992

A. Hepatosplenomegaly
B. Low haemoglobin
C. Low reticulocyte count
D. Hypercellular bone marrow
E. Normal platelet count

398. The absolute contraindication of phototherapy is : AIIMS 1985, 96

A. Hereditary spherocytosis
B. Idiopathic thrombocytopenic purpura
C. Severe Rh incompatibility
D. Severe ABO incompatibility

399. Aminocaproic acid would be recommended for a hemophilic child with: AIIMS 1991

A. Epistaxis
B. Haematuria
C. Oral bleeding
D. Hamarthrosis

400. What is the role of corticosteroid in the management of idiopathic thrombocytopenic purpura ? Bihar 1991

A. Prevent progression to pancytopenia
B. Prevent C N S haemorrhage
C. Prevent fatal exsanguination
D. Reduce spleen size

401. All these features suggest acute non-lymphocytic leukaemia except : AIIMS 1999

A. Presence of periorbital swelling with proptosis (chloroma)
B. Gingival hyperplasia
C. Blasts are peroxidase negative
D. Features of disseminated intravascular coagulation present

402. Most frequent cause of neonatal thrombocytopenic purpura is : AIIMS 1993

A. Infection
B. Drug idiosyncrasy
C. Erythroblastosis
D. Large haemangiomas

403. The following conditions are associated with hypochromic microcytic anaemia except : AMU 1997

A. Iron deficiency
B. B6 deficiency
C. Vit. C deficiency
D. Thalassemia major

404. The type of blood to use if time does not permit adequate cross matching in an emergency is : AMU 1995

A. O, Rh negative
B. O, Rh positive
C. B, Rh positive
D. A, Rh negative

Ans. 397. C 398. B 399. C 400. B 401. C 402. A
403. C 404. A

405. Physiologic anemia of newborn is most severe at the age of : **Rohtak 1999**

A. 4 months B. 2 months
C. 4 weeks D. 2 weeks

406. Paroxsymal haemoglobinuria is associated with : **AMC 1991**

A. Syphilis B. Chloromycetin toxicity
C. Mongolism D. Ingestion of lead

407. Commonest cause of anemia during childhood is : **AMC 1991**

A. Vitamin B12 deficiency B. Folic acid deficiency
C. Pyridoxine deficiency D. Iron deficiency

408. Characteristic features of acute lymphoblastic leukaemia include : **AIIMS 1996**

A. Tumour cells which react with antisera raised against B lymphocytes.
B. Better prognosis when the white cell count at presentation is very high.
C. Massive splenomegaly.
D. Spread to the meninges unless prophylactic treatment to the central nervous system is given.

409. Prednisone is the treatment of choice in a haemophiliac with : **AMU 1998**

A. Spontaneous haematuria
B. Gingival bleeding
C. Traumatic hemarthrosis
D. None of the above

410. In hemophilia, which of the following is abnormal : **DNB 1993**

A. BT B. PT
C. PTT D. None of the above

411. Poor prognosis in acute lymphatic leukaemia is indicated by all, except: **UPSC 1999**

A. Intrathoracic mass B. Children between 2 & 10 years
C. Cranial secondaries D. WBC around 10000/mm

412. Haemorrhagic disease of the newborn most commonly appears in : **AP 1999**

A. Haemophilic diseased infants
B. Thrombocytopenic infants
C. Breast-fed infants
D. Early artificial milk-fed infants

413. Hereditary spherocytosis is : **AIIMS 1983, 94**

A. Autosomal dominant B. Autosomal recessive
C. Sex-linked recessive D. Sex-linked dominant

Ans. 405. B 406. D 407. D 408. D 409. A 410. C
411. D 412. C 413. A

414. Bronze baby syndrome is a complication of : AIIMS 1984, 96

A. ABO incompatibility B. Rh incompatibility
C. Chloromycetin toxicity D. Phototherapy

415. True about spherocytosis is all of the following except: AIIMS 1984, 96

A. Gall stones
B. Positive Coomb's test suggests immuno-hemolytic anaemia
C. Splenomegaly
D. ↑ MCH and MCHC

416. Serum iron is raised in : AIIMS 1995

A. Chronic renal failure B. Thalassemia
C. Iron deficiency anaemia D. Viral hepatitis

417. A 6-year-old child with petechiae, most commonly has: AIIMS 1983; UPSC 1994

A. Leukaemia
B. Scurvy
C. Idiopathic thrombocytic purpura
D. Aplastic anaemia

418. Which of the following is not seen in aplastic anaemia: AIIMS 1985; PGI 1995

A. Anaemia B. Purpura
C. Haemorrhage D. Splenomegaly

419. In-G-6-P-D deficiency, RBC's hemolysis is induced by: AIIMS 1986, 88; PGI 1990

A. Erythromycin B. Dapsone
C. Chloromycetin D. Levamisol

420. True about idiopathic thrombocytopenic purpura is : AIIMS 1986; UPSC 1996

A. It is diagnosed by poor clot retraction
B. Splenomegaly is present in a majority
C. Remits of its own without any treatment in all
D. Decrease in number of megakaryocytes in bone marrow

421. Sideroblastic anaemia may be caused by all of the following except : AIIMS 1996

A. Lead poisoning B. Collagen-vascular disease
C. Cutaneous porphyria D. Iron deficiency

422. Which of the following drug may be useful in agranulocytosis : DNB 1992

A. Cyclosporine B. Azathioprin
C. Lithium D. ACTH

Ans. 414. D 415. D 416. B 417. C 418. D 419. B
420. C 421. C 422. C

423. Pancytopenia is associated with : **AIIMS 1987, 90**
A. PNH (Paroxysmal Nocturnal hemoglybinuria)
B. Paroxysmal cold hemoglobinuria
C. Thalassemia
D. Hereditary spherocytosis

424. Haemolytic uremic syndrome in children is not associated with : **UPSC 1996**
A. Changes in the shape of the R.B.C. (Burr cells)
B. Thrombocytopenia
C. Essential changes involving venous inflammation and subsequent thrombosis
D. Severe haemolytic anaemia

425. Treatment of acute lymphoblastic leukaemia in child with CNS manifestations is : **AIIMS 1988; UPSC 1991**
A. Intrathecal methotrexate
B. Vincristine and prednisolone
C. Intrathecal vincristine
D. Intrathecal steroids and vincristine

426. Regarding hereditary spherocytosis, true is : **AIIMS 1990**
A. ↓ Osmotic fragility
B. Enzyme deficiency present
C. Choice of Treatment-Splenectomy
D. Moderate splenomegaly found

427. Palpable purpura is seen in all except : **AIIMS 1990**
A. ITP
B. Drug induced
C. Mixed essential cyroglobulinemia
D. Vasculitis

428. Majority of chronic lymphocytic leukemia is of type : **PGI 1986; AIIMS 1996**
A. T-cell
B. B-cell
C. Null cell
D. Mixed B-cell and T-cell

429. Haemoglobin F is : **PGI 1998**
A. $\alpha_2\beta_2$
B. $\alpha_2\gamma_2$
C. $\alpha_2\delta_2$
D. $\alpha_1\beta_1$

430. 'Warm' type of hermolytic anaemia is caused by all except : **PGI 1994**
A. Mycoplasma
B. Methyldopa
C. Leukemia (chronic lymphatics)
D. Hodgkin's lymphoma
E. SLE

Ans. **423. A** **424. C** **425. A** **426. C** **427. A** **428. B**
429. B **430. A**

431. Iron deficiency anaemia in children is characterised by all of the following except : UPSC 1996

A. Microcytic hypochromic red cell morphology
B. Decreased serum ferritin
C. Decreased iron binding capacity
D. Decreased serum iron levels

432. Disseminated intravascular coagulation is common in: PGI 1998

A. Acute lymphocytic leukaemia
B. Acute myelocytic leukaemia
C. CML (chronic myeloid leukaemia)
D. CLL (chronic lymphocytic leukaemia)
E. None of the above

433. Increased fetal Hb is seen in : AIIMS 1997

A. Juvenile CML
B. Pure red cell aplasia
C. Hereditary Spherocytosis
D. Polycythemia vera

434. In Erythroblastosis fetalis not involved is : AIIMS 1997

A. Anti C
B. D
C. E
D. Anti Lewis

435. Microcytic Hypochromic blood picture is not seen in : AIIMS 1997

A. Thalassemia Major
B. Thalassemia Minor
C. Iron deficiency anemia
D. Fanconi's anemia

436. A 2-year old healthy child is brought with history of accidental ingestion of some tablets. He is cyanosed but without any respiratory distress. The most likely diagnosis is : UPSC 1997

A. Polycythemia
B. Methemoglobinemia
C. Haemoglobinemia
D. Congenital cyanotic heart disease

437. True about Henoch Schonlein purpura is following except : PGI 1984, 85, 90

A. Purpura on lower limb
B. Arthritis
C. Thromboembolism
D. Hematuria
E. Anemia

438. Dactylitis is seen in : UPSC 1999

A. ITP
B. Sickle cell anemia
C. HbD disease
D. Alpha thalasemia
E. Aplastic anemia

Ans. **431. C** **432. B** **433. A** **434. D** **435. D** **436. B** **437. C** **438. B**

439. Consider the following statements : **CSE 1997**

Tolerance of infants to blood loss is poor because :

1. A small amount of lost blood represents a sizeable fraction of cardiac output.
2. Of poor defence mechanism to blood loss as the peripheral circulatory resistance is high.
3. Of ineffective vasoconstriction of peripheral vessels.

Of these statements :

A. 1, 2 and 3 are correct B. 1 and 2 are correct
C. 2 and 3 are correct D. 1 and 3 are correct

440. Foetal acidosis is pH less than : **Rajasthan 1998**

A. 7.0 B. 7.2
C. 7.3 D. 7.4

441. A 9-year old child has pallor, fever, pain all over the body. CNS examination and hemogram are normal. GPE shows proptosis. Diagnosis is :
AIIMS 1983, 85; UPSC 1986; ESI 1999

A. Purpura
B. Leukaemia
C. Neuroblastoma
D. Cavernous sinus thrombosis

442. Treatment of choice in child with Hb-5 gm %, anisocytosis, poikilocytosis and hypochromic microcytic picture is : **Delhi 1993**

A. Iron dextran B. Blood transfusion
C. Packed cells D. Oral iron therapy

443. Punctate basophilia with anaemia is seen in :
UPSC 1987, JIPMER 1992

A. PEM B. Lead poisoning
C. Measles D. Aspirin poisoning

444. In Hemochromatosis, iron accumulates maximally in :
AIIMS 1986, JIPMER 1992

A. Bone B. Kidneys
C. Liver D. Spleen

445. Following are true of childhood ITP except :
UPSC 1987, AIIMS 1992

A. Prolonged clotting time
B. Preceding viral infection
C. Decreased bone marrow megakaryocytes
D. Splenectomy for chronic cases

Ans. 439. A 440. B 441. C 442. C 443. B 444. C
445. C

446. If a one year old on breast milk, develops severe pallor with hepatomegaly but no splenomegaly, the investigation of choice would be : AIIMS 1992
A. Serum iron estimation
B. Fetal Hb estimation
C. Serum Vit B_{12} level
D. Serum folic acid level

447. The opportunistic infection most commonly seen in children with neutropenia is : JIPMER 1993
A. Staphylococcal
B. Pneumococcal
C. Streptococcal
D. Gram negative rods

448. The Hb to appear first in the fetus is : TN 1993
A. HbA
B. HbA_2
C. HbF
D. Hb Gower

449. The major site of active haemopoesis in a foetus of 5 months is : TN 1993
A. Spleen
B. Liver
C. Lymph nodes
D. Bone marrow

450. The percentage of foetal haemoglobin at birth is : Bihar 1999
A. 90%
B. 20%
C. 70%
D. 100%

451. Megaloblastic anaemia is most likely to occur in infant being fed : PGI 1986
A. Goat's milk
B. Soya formulae
C. Human milk
D. Cereals before 6 months

452. Large doses of Vitamin-K administered to a new-born may result in : AIIMS 1992
A. Hypothyroidism
B. RBC destruction
C. Bulging of fontanelles
D. Prolonged bilirubinemia

453. Bone marrow transplantation is not indicated in : AP 1993
A. Sickle cell anaemia
B. Multiple myeloma
C. Leukaemia
D. Metastasis

454. Philadelphia chromosome is : AP 1993
A. t (8; 22)
B. t (8; 21)
C. t (15; 17)
D. t (8; 14)

455. Sickling of red blood cells occurs in : PGI 1993
A. Eight per cent of whites
B. Megaloblastic anemia
C. Only in sickle cell anemia, not sickle cell trait
D. Thalassemia and sickle cell trait occurring together

456. Absolute lymphocytosis occurs in all except : AIIMS 1984, 95
A. Mumps
B. Whooping cough
C. Enteric fever
D. Infectious mononucleosis

Ans. **446. A** **447. A** **448. C** **449. B** **450. C** **451. A**
452. D **453. A** **454. A** **455. D** **456. C**

457. In alpha-thalassemia, HbH is formed by chains of ——: **DNB 1990**

A. α_3, β_1
B. α_4
C. α_1, β_3
D. β_4

458. The commonest cause of aplastic anaemia is : **AIIMS 1979, 93**

A. Idiopathic
B. Chloramphenicol
C. Phenylbutazone
D. Petroleum products

459. Normal infant has ——— mg of iron at the time of birth: **DNB 1991**

A. 100—200
B. 250—300
C. 500—600
D. 900—1000

460. The following are the correct facts in relation to hemorrhage disease of new born except : **Karnataka 1999**

A. Self-limited bleeding disorder
B. Results from deficiency of coagulation factors dependent on Vitamin-K
C. More common in formula fed infants
D. In most cases, hemorrhagic manifestations become evident for the 2nd and 3rd day of life

461. Autoimmune hemolytic anaemia is seen in : **AIIMS 1994**

A. AML
B. CLL
C. Multiple myeloma
D. Sickle anaemia

462. All of the following are true for sickle cell anaemia except : **AIIMS 1994**

A. Leukopenia
B. Enlarged heart
C. Fish vertebra
D. Pulmonary arterial hypertension

463. In children, disseminated intravascular coagulation is associated with: **UPSC 1994**

A. Thrombocytopaenia
B. Normal thrombin time
C. Polycythemia
D. Generalised or fulminant gram negative septicaemia

464. All of the following are known complications of neonatal polycythemia except : **UPSC 1994**

A. Renal vein thrombosis
B. Hyperbilirubinaemia
C. Necrotising enterocolitis
D. Hyaline membrane disease

Ans. **457. D** **458. A** **459. B** **460. C** **461. B** **462. A**
463. D **464. C**

465. Which of the following are poor prognostic factors in acute lymphoblastic leukemia in children : UPSC 1994

A.. Total below 2 years

B. Total leucocyte count above 25,000/cu mm

C. Central nervous system involvement

D. Null cell type leukaemia

466. Juvenile myeloid leukemia is associated with all except : AI 1994

A. Philadelphia chromosome

B. Significant lymphadenopathy

C. Marked pallor

D. Raised fetal hemoglobin

467. Polycythemia in infants will cause the following except: AI 1994

A. Increased physiological jaundice

B. Cerebral ischemia

C. CHF

D. Vitamin-E related anemia

468. Henoch Schonlein Purpura is characterized by all except : AI 1994

A. Thrombocytopenia

B. Arthralgia

C. Glomerulonephritis

D. Abdominal pain

469. The beta thalasemia (Homozygotic), is characterized by all except : AIIMS 1986, 87; AI 1994

A. Increased HbA2

B. Increased HbF

C. ↑ Adult Hb

D. Reduced haematocrit

470. Commonest haematological malignancy in children is: Kerala 1994

A. CLL

B. CML

C. AML

D. ALL

471. Indication for exchange transfusion at birth is : Delhi 1995

A. Cord Hb < 16 gm%

B. Cord bilirubin —3 mg%

C. Cord bilirubin —5 mg%

D. Mother antibody titre > 1 : 64

472. A five-year old child is brought with fever and pallor. On examination he is found to have anaemia, petechial haemorrhages, lymphadenopathy, tenderness of the bones and hepatosplenomegaly. The most likely diagnosis is : UPSC 1995

A. Acute rheumatic fever

B. Infectious mononucleosis

C. Idiopathic thrombocytopenic purpura

D. Acute leukaemia

Ans. **465. C** **466. A** **467. D** **468. A** **469. C** **470. D**
471. C **472. D**

473. In newborn baby, thrombocytopenia is caused by : AIIMS 1999

A. ABO incompatibility
B. Isoimmune thrombocytopenia
C. Auto-immune thrombocytopenia purpura
D. SLE

474. An infant with history of diarrhoea, 5 days back has urea 200 mg% and creatinine 5 mg%. The platelet count is 9,0000. Fragmented RBC's are found in the peripheral smear. The most possible diagnosis is : AIIMS 1999

A. HUS
B. DIS
C. Microangiopathic hemolytic anemia
D. Porphyria

475. A 4 year old child presented with anemia and splenomegaly. Blood smear showed target cells. There is similar history in the family. The best investigation is: AIIMS 1999, 2001; AI 2001

A. Hemoglobin electrophoresis
B. Osmotic fragility
C. Corrected reticulocyte count > 25%
D. Osmotic fragility of RBC's

476. Coomb's positive hemolytic anemia occurs in : PGI 1999

A. SLE
B. ITP
C. CML
D. Rifampicin intake

477. 6 months old baby with severe pallor and hepatosplenomegaly. Similiar history with the sibling. Investigation of choice is : TN 1999

A. Bone marrow biopsy
B. Hb. electrophoresis
C. Hb. estimation
D. Platelet count

478. Fetal Hb equals adult Hb at : TN 1999

A. At Birth
B. 2 months
C. 4 months
D. 6 months

479. Serum Iron level in child -------- mgm: TN 1999

A. 20-50
B. 100-200
C. 50-100
D. 200 - 350

480. The following laboratory parameter does not carry a bad prognosis in acute lymphocytic leukaemia : AIIMS 1990

A. Presence of anaemia
B. Low initial platelet count
C. Initial WBC count more than 1 lakh/cubic mm
D. L_2 cell morphology

Ans. 473. B 474. A 475. A 476. A 477. A 478. B 479. D 480. A

481. All are seen in juvenile CML except : Kerala 1999
A. Thrombocytopenia B. Monocytosis
C. ↑ fetal Hb D. Ph chromosome

482. Drug of choice in the treatment of idiopathic thrombocytopenic purpura is : Rohtak 1997
A. Oestrogen B. Nitrogen mustard
C. Amethopterin D. Corticosteroids

483. Acute idiopathic thrombocytopenic purpura can follow: AIIMS 1991
A. Mumps B. Rubella
C. Chickenpox D. All of the above

484. During the process of coagulation, the platelets release—which promotes vasoconstriction : AIIMS 1991
A. Serotonin B. Fibrinogen
C. Thromboplastin D. Hyaluronidase

485. The bone marrow in idiopathic thrombocytopenic purpura on examination, exhibits : AIIMS 1993
A. Foam cells
B. Aplasia of all elements
C. Absence of megakaryoctes
D. Normal or increased number of megakaryocytes

486. A leukaemoid reaction with a predominance of lymphocytes occurs in : AMU 1997
A. Chicken pox B. Leukaemia
C. Ulcerative colitis D. Acute tuberculosis

487. Peak age of idiopathic thrombocytopenic purpura is ——— years : DNB 1990
A. 1—3 B. 2—8
C. 8—12 D. 12—16

488. In ABO hemolytic disease of the newborn direct Coomb's test is : UPSC 1984, 87
A. Usually negative
B. Usually mild positive
C. Usually strongly positive
D. Positive in cases where peripheral smear shows microspherocytosis

489. O+ve mother delivers A-ve baby. Which of the following blood will be ideal if the baby needs exchange blood transfusion ? Rohtak 1984, 97
A. O -ve B. A +ve
C. A -ve D. O -ve cells suspended in AB plasma

Ans. **481. D** **482. D** **483. D** **484. A** **485. D** **486. A**
487. B **488. A** **489. D**

490. A 5 year old girl came with history of progressively increasing pallor since birth and hepatosplenomegaly. Which of the following is the most relevant test for achieving diagnosis : AI 2004

A. Hb electrophoresis B. Peripheral smear examination
C. Osmotic fragility test D. Bone marrow examination

491. A 5 year old child presents with history of fever off and on for past 2 weeks and petechial spots all over the body and increasing pallor for past 1 month. Examination reveals splenomegaly of 2 cms below costal margin. The most likely diagnosis is : AI 2004

A. Acute leukemia
B. Idiopathic thrombocytopenic purpura
C. Hypersplenism
D. Aplastic anaemia

492. A nine month old boy of Sindhi parents presented to you with complaints of progressive lethargy, irritability and pallor since 6 months of age. Examination revealed severe Pallor. Investigations showed Hb- 3.8 gm%, MCV - 58 fl, MCH - 19.4 pg/cell. Blood film shows osmotic fragility is normal (target cells and normoblasts). X-ray skull shows expansion of erythroid marrow. Which of the following is the most likely diagnosis: AI 2004

A. Iron deficiency anaemia
B. Acute lymphoblastic anaemia
C. Hemoglobin D disease
D. Hereditary spherocytosis

493. Treatment of choice for Thalassemia Major is : UPSC 2004

A. Blood transfusion and iron therapy
B. Folic acid and desferrioxamine
C. Blood transfusion and desferrioxamine
D. Iron, blood transfusion and desferrioxamine

494. When does switch over from fetal to adult hemoglobin synthesis begin : AI 2005

A. 14 weeks gestation B. 30 weeks gestation
C. 36 weeks gestation D. 7-10 days postnatal

495. The most common leukocytoclastic vasculitis affecting children is : AI 2005

A. Takayasu disease
B. Mucocutaneous lymph node syndrome (Kawasaki disease)
C. Henoch Schonelin purpura
D. Polyarteritis nodosa

Ans. 490. D 491. A 492. C 493. C 494. A 495. C

EXPLANATIONS OF CLINICAL ASPECTS

1. Ans.— C. Is normal after glycol ingestion
2. Ans.— C. Cholera

   High-anion gap metabolic acidosis is seen in lactic acidosis, ketoacidosis (diabetic, alcoholic, starvation), toxins (ethylene glycol, methanol, salicylates), renal failure acute or chronic).
3. Ans.— A. Ketoacidosis
4. Ans.— C. Hyperkalemia
5. Ans.— B. 20 : 1
6. Ans.— A. Deep and sighing
7. Ans.— A. Hypochloremic hyponatremic alkalosis
8. Ans.— C. Mannitol
9. Ans.— A. Kussmaul's breathing
10. Ans.— D. Thrombocytopenia
11. Ans.— C. Respiration does not effectively control metabolic alkalosis
12. Ans.— A. Acute pancreatitis
13. Ans.— A. Quinine

    Hyperglycemia is caused by asparaginase, chlorthalidone, diazoxide, encainide, ethacrynic acid, furosemide, glucocorticoids, GH, HIV-protease inhibitor, niacin, OCPs, phenytoin, pentamidine, thiazides, Hypoglycemia is cause by ACE inhibitor, insulin, octreotide, oral hypoglycemics, pentamidine and quinine.
14. Ans.— B. 154 meq
15. Ans.— B. 15-25%
16. Ans.— B. Seen with primary hyperparathyroidism

    It is seen with hypoparathyroidism.
17. Ans.— B. ↑ reflex

18. Ans.— B. Chronic renal failure

19. Ans.— B. Rebound hypoglycemia

20. Ans.— A. Reual tubular acidosis

Non-anion gap acidosis is seen in —GI bicarbonate loss (diarrhoea ext. pancreatic or bowel drainage, ureterosigmoidostomy, jejunal or ileal loop, drugs — calcium chloride, magnesium sulfate, cholestyramine), Renal acidosis (hypokalemia, hyperkalemia), drug induced hyperkalemia (potassium sparing diuretics, trimethoprim, pentamidine, ACE inhibitors, Nonsteroidal antiinflammatory drugs, cyclosporic, others - Acid increase (Ammonium chloride hyperalimentation, ketosis with ketone excretion, rapid saline administration, Hippurate, cation exchange resins).

21. Ans.— C. Altered sensorium

22. Ans.— C. Hyperkalemia

23. Ans.— E. Oral administration of orange juice

24. Ans.— E. None of the above

25. Ans.— E. Addison's disease

26. Ans.— B. Oliguric phase of acute renal failure

In this phase, hyperkalemia is seen.

27. Ans.— B. Urinary sodium excretion

28. Ans.— D. Lisonopril

Hypokalemia is caused by alkali induced alkalosis, amphotericin-B, carbenoxolone, corticosteroids, diuretics, gentamicin, insulin, laxatives (abused), mineralo-corticoids, some glucocorticoids, osmotic diuretics, sympathomimetic agents, tetracycline, theophylline, and vitamin B-12.

29. Ans.— E. Novobiocin

30. Ans.— C. Respiratory alkalosis

31. Ans.— B. QRS prolongation

Lithium, thiazides, aluminium intoxication, vitamin-A intoxication, immobilization, hyper-thyroidism, leukemia, lymphoma, kidney tumor, metastasis may also produce this.

32. Ans.— All

33. Ans.— D. Sinus bradycardia

34. Ans.— C. Abdominal distension

35. Ans.— C. Increased bowel sounds

36. Ans.— C. Salicylate poisoning

Respiratory alkalosis is seen early in the course of poisoning and lactic and ketoacidosis in later stages.

37. Ans.— B. Haemodialysis

38. Ans.— D. Tomato

39. Ans.— B. Respiratory alkalosis

The causes of Tetany includes: malabsorption, osteomalacia, Hypoparathyroidism. Excessive vomiting, excessive oral alkali, Hyperventilation, Pri. hyper-aldosteronism.

40. Ans.— C. Raised potassium

41. Ans.— D. Hepatic coma

42. Ans.— B. Pylorus

43. Ans.— D. Hypercalcuria

44. Ans.— A. Severe pyloric stenosis for 2 hours

45. Ans.— B. Increased potassium loss

46. Ans.— C. It diminishes deep tendon reflexes

47. Ans.— D. Corticosteroid therapy

48. Ans.— A. Resp. alkalosis

49. Ans.— A. SIADH

50. Ans.— C. I/V ringer lactate

51. Ans.— A. Acute tubular necrosis

52. Ans.— D. $NaHCO_3$

53. Ans.— A. HCO_3 decreased

54. Ans.— B. Gout

Hypercalcemia is seen in primary hyperpara-thyroidism, lithium therapy, familial hypocalciuric hypercalcemia, malignancy related (Ca breast with metastasis, Ca lung and kidney with humeral mediation), multiple myeloma, leukemia, lymphoma, vitamin-D intoxication, sarcoidosis and other granulomatous disease, idiopathic hypercalcemia of infancy, hyperthyroidism, immobilization, thiazides, vitamin-A intoxication, associated with renal failure (severe secondary hyperpara-thyroidism, aluminium intoxication and milk alkali syndrome).

55. Ans.— D. Sickle cell crisis

56. Ans.— A. 55 mmol/L

57. Ans.— B. Metabolic alkalosis

58. Ans.— C. Periodic paralysis

59. Ans.— D. Phenytoin therapy

60. Ans.— B. Hypokalemia

61. Ans.— C. Prolonged QT

62. Ans.— D. 1, 2 and 4 are correct

Hyponatremia may also be due to drugs due to dilutional (antipsycholies, carbamazepine, chlorpropamide, cyclophosphamide, desmopressin, diuretics, intravenous immunoglobulin, (octreotide, SSRI's, Vincristine) and salt wasting (diuretics, enemas and mannitol).

63. Ans.— C. Hyperkalemia

64. Ans.— A. Shortened QT interval

65. Ans.— A. Hyponatremia

66. Ans.— C. Potassium

67. Ans.— C. 130

68. Ans.— A. Bicarbonate

69. Ans.— A. Proximal S_1

70. Ans.— C. Respiratory alkalosis

71. Ans.— A. CO_2 inhalation

72. Ans.— B. Ringer Lartate

73. Ans.— B. 4 3 1 2

74. Ans.— D. Respiratory acidosis with decompensated metabolic acidosis

75. Ans.— D. Normal saline

76. Ans.— A. Diabetic ketoacidosis

77. Ans.— D. Single left coronary artery stenosis

78. Ans.— B. Metabolic acidosis

79. Ans.— A. Myxoedema

80. Ans.— A. Cong. hypertrophic pyloric stenosis

81. Ans.— B. Patient hypoventilates

82. Ans.— A. Diabetes mellitus

83. Ans.— B. Profuse sweating

84. Ans.— C. Diarrhoea

85. Ans.— D. Na would return to previous level spontaneously on correction of blood glucose
Glucose helps in restoration of Na levels.

86. Ans.— D. Metabolic acidosis and respiratory acidosis

87. Ans.— C. Metabolic acidosis

88. Ans.— All

89. Ans.— D. Ureterosigmoidostomy

90. Ans.— C. Shortening of Q-T interval in ECG
Hypocalcemia - leads :
* QT - Prolongation
* Chavestak, sign (Tapping Myokyemia) + ve
* Trosseua's sign (Carpopedal Spasm on cuff-Inflation at arm.)

91. Ans.— D. Acidosis leads to movement of potassium from extra-cellular to intracellular fluid compartment

92. Ans.— A. Cholera

93. Ans.— A. Mineralocorticoid deficiency

94. Ans.— A. 250 mEq

95. Ans.— A. Congenital hypertrophic pyloric stenosis
* K^+ Major Intracellular ion
* K+ Conc. - 3 - 5 m Eq/l L in plasma
* In Metabolic acidosis 60% of H+ load is buffered inside the cell to maintain Electro negativity it must be accompanied by an anion exchange for Intra-cellular K+. Thus it is leading to Hyperkalemia."

Causes of High anion Gap metabolic acidosis :-
* Lactic acidosis (types A & B)
* Ketoacidosis - (Diabetic, Alcoholic, starvation)
* Toxins - (Ethylene glycol, Methanol, salicylates)
* Renal failure (acute or chronic)

Acidosis (normal Anion gap)
A. Diarrhea
B. External panereatic fistula
C. Urterosigmoidostomy
D. Proximal RTA
E. Mineralocorticoid deficiency

Causes of Metabolic alkalosis :-

- **Acute alkali administration**
- **Milk alkali syndrome**
- **Vomiting**
- **Diuretics**
- **Bartter's syndrome**
- **Estrogen therapy (thiazide therapy)**
- **Primary aldosteronism**
- **11β hydroxylase deficiency**
- **17α hydroxylase deficiency**
- **Cushing's syndrome**
- **Formula : - X = 0.3 x base excess x body weight and base supply = 1/3 to 1/2 of X.**
- **So X = 0.3 x 50 x 30 = 450 mEq.**
- **So base supply will be between 150 to 225.**
- **So most appropriate answer here would be A (most suitable)**

96. Ans.— D. Siggard-Andersen nomogram

- **Use of the Siggard–Andersen curve nomogram to plot the acid base characteristic of arterial blood is helpful in clinical situations.**
- **This nomogram has PCO_2 plotted on a log scale on the vertical axis and pH on horizontal axis.**
- **Any point to the left of vertical line through pH 7.40 indicates acidosis, and any point to the right indicates alkalosis.**
- **The position of the point above or below the horizontal line through a PCO_2 of 40 mmHg defines the effective degree of hypoventilation of hyperventilation.**

Note:

The magnitude of the membrane potential at any given time depends upon the distribution of Na^+, K^+ and Cl^- and the permeability of membrane to each of these ions which described by Goldman constant field equation.

97. Ans.— B. **Tumor lysis syndrome**

Tumor lysis syndrome is a well-recognized clinical entity that is characterized by various combinations of hyperuricemia, hyperkalemia, hyperphos-phatemia, lactic acidosis, and hypocalcemia and is caused by the destruction of a large number of rapidly failure develops as a result of the syndrome.

Tumor lysis syndrome is most frequently associated with the treatment of Burkitt's lymphoma, acute lymphomas, but it also may be seen with chronic leukemias and rarely, with solid tumors. This syndrome has been seen in patients with chronic lymphocytic leukemia after treatment with fludarabine and cladribine. Tumor lysis syndrome usually occurs during or shortly (1 to 5 days) after malignancies causes tumor lysis syndrome.

98. Ans.— A. **Normal prothrombin time**

The disorder is characterised by a reduced level of vWF which is often accompanied by a secondary reduction in factor VIII & prolongation in the bleeding time. The gene for vWF is located on chromosome 12 & therefore the disorder is inherited as an autosomal dominant.

99. Ans.— D. Hematuria

100. Ans.— D. IV infusion

101. Ans.— B. A_2G_2

102. Ans.— C. Infants fed on goats milk

103. Ans.— A. ↑ Factor-X

104. Ans.— C. ↓ Fibrinolytic activity

105. Ans.— B. Reduced iron levels

106. Ans.— C. Thrombocytopenia

107. Ans.— B. Hypothyroidism

108. Ans.— D. 40,000

109. Ans.— B. Acute lymphoblastic leukaemia

110. Ans.— C. Severe skin lesions

Features of A.I. Porphyria are—no skin lesions, abdominal pain, Neuropsychiatric symptoms, delirium. Attack is triggered by barbiturates, oestrogens, Griseofulvin, sulphonamides.

111. Ans.— C. Liver disease
112. Ans.— D. Leukemoid reaction
113. Ans.— D. Polycythemia vera
114. Ans.— D. Congestive cardiac failure
115. Ans.— C. Severe anaemia
116. Ans.— D. WBC around 10,000/mm^3
117. Ans.— C. Myocardial infarction
118. Ans.— B. Intracellular crystals
119. Ans.— D. AHG deficiency
120. Ans.— A. Henoch-Schonlein purpura
121. Ans.— B. 5th-8th day
122. Ans.— B. Gaucher's disease
123. Ans.— A. Gastric malignancy
124. Ans.— B. Philadelphia chromosome
125. Ans.— A. Auer rods in blast sells
126. Ans.— B. Busulfan
127. Ans.— C. Splenic infarction
128. Ans.— A. Both A and R are true and R is the correct explanation of A
129. Ans.— B. Erythroid hypoplasia of the marrow
130. Ans.— D. Microangiopathic haemolytic anaemia
131. Ans.— A. Decreased oxygen affinity
132. Ans.— B. Amino acids
133. Ans.— B. A contractile protein
134. Ans.— B. B-cell
135. Ans.— A. HbS B Glu-Val
136. Ans.— A. HLA A_3
137. Ans.— D. All of the above
138. Ans.— C. Bone marrow failure
139. Ans.— A. 1, 2 and 3 are correct
140. Ans.— A. I (i), II (ii) III (iii) IV (iv)
141. Ans.— B. Increased RBC osmotic fragility
142. Ans.— B Petechia are frequently present

Thrombocytopenia is caused by 3 mechanisms: decreased BM production, increased splenic seqestration or accidental destruction of platelets.

143. Ans.— A. 0.6%

144. Ans.— C. Thalassemia

145. Ans.— A. Disseminated intravascular coagulation

146. Ans.— D. Decreased platelet count

147. Ans.— D. Acquired membrane defect

148. Ans.— A. Cloxacillin

Agranulocytosis is produced by aprindine, Captopril, carbimazole, cefotaxine, Chloramphenicol, Clozapine, cotrimoxazole, Cytotoxics, gold salts, indomethacin, methimazole, oxyphenbutazone, phenothiazines, phenylbutazone, propylthiouracil, sulfonamides, ticlopidine, tolbutamide, tricyclic antidepressants.

149. Ans.— E. All of the above

In G-6-P-D deficiency, antimalarials (primaquine, pamaquine, dapsone), sulfonamides (sulfamethoxa-zole), nitrofurantoin, analgesics (acetanilid), vitamin-K, doxorubicin, methylene blue, nalidixic acid, furazolidone, niridazole, phenazopyridine are contraindicated.

150. Ans.— A. Amoebic hepatitis

Eosinophilia can be caused by drugs - aspirin, chlorpropamide, EM imipramine L-tryptophan, methotrexate montelukast, nitrofurantoin, procarbazine, sulfas, zafirlukast.

151. Ans.— D. Systemic lupus erythematosus

G-CSF is not commonly used but is reserved for management of certain forms of neutropenia due to depressed production especially that related to cancer chemotherapy.

152. Ans.— B. Sideroblastic anaemia

153. Ans.— D. 120 days

154. Ans.— E. In pyogenic infections

155. Ans.— D. Appearance of lymphadenopathy

156. Ans.— E. Normal arterial oxygen tension

157. Ans.— C. Increased osmotic fragility

158. Ans.— A. Globulin

159. Ans.— B. Multiple myeloma

In multiple myeloma, ESR is markedly increased.

160. **Ans.— A. Hemolytic anemia**

161. **Ans.— D. Retroperitonial lymphadenopathy**

Pain is the most common symptom of multiple myelomainvolving back and ribs

162. **Ans.— C. Endothelial dysintegrity**

163. **Ans.— B. Von Willebrand's disease**

164. **Ans.— D. Chorea**

165. **Ans.— B. Thrombocytosis**

166. **Ans.— B. Sickle cell anemia**

167. **Ans.— C. Hookworm infestation**

168. **Ans.— B. Hypothalamus**

169. **Ans.— B. Herediatary spherocytosis**

170. **Ans.— A. Serum B_{12}**

171. **Ans.— C. MCHC low**

172. **Ans.— B. Breast Ca**

Causes of DIC—

(a) Infection—E coli, N meningococci, streptococcus pneumonia, Malaria

(b) Obstetric—Abrupto placenta, Retained dead fetus, pre-eclampsia, Amniotic fluid embolism

(c) Cancer—Lung, Pancreas, prostate.

173. **Ans.— C. Neutrophil alkaline phosphatase is very low**

174. **Ans.— C. Cold antibody haemolytic anemia**

175. **Ans.— D. Indicates levels of glucose in blood**

176. **Ans.— B. Decreased serum ferritin**

177. **Ans.— B. Cyclophosphamide**

178. **Ans.— D. XII**

179. **Ans.— B. Antithrombin-III**

180. **Ans.— C. IX**

181. **Ans.— B. Increased megakaryocytes with non-budding appearance**

182. **Ans.— B. V**

183. **Ans.— C. 10 days**

184. **Ans.— C. 3-4 days**

185. **Ans.— D. Shigellosis**

186. Ans.— C. 1 mg

187. Ans.— B. Microcytosis

188. Ans.— C. Megaloblastic anemia

189. Ans.— A. 2 days

190. Ans.— C. Haemoglobin-A2

191. Ans.— A. Oxymethalone

192. Ans.— A. Weekly venesection

193. Ans.— D. Thrombocytopenia

194. Ans.— D. Increased osmotic fragility

195. Ans.— B. +2 to +6°C

196. Ans.— B. Bone

197. Ans.— C. Coproporphyrin

198. Ans.— C. Myeloid metaplasia

199. Ans.— B. Chediak-Higashi syndrome

200. Ans.— D. Bone marrow aspiration

201. Ans.— D. Cataract

202. Ans.— D. Bilirubinuria

Hemolytic anaemia can be caused by drugs— Aminosolicyclic acid, cephalosporins chlorproma-zine, dapsone, insulin, INH, Levodopa, Mefenamic acid, melphalan, methyldopa, penicillins, phenacetin, procainamide, Quinidine, Rifampicin, sulfonamides.

203. Ans.— B. Normal arterial oxygen suturation

204. Ans.— D. Samples should be preserved in a cool environment

205. Ans.— B. Haemolytic anaemia

206. Ans.— B. Normocytic normochromic blood picture

207. Ans.— A. Thrombocytopenia

208. Ans.— C. Protoporphyrin-III

209. Ans.— C. Henoch-Schonlein's purpura

It is a reactive vasculitis and IgA is raised.

210. Ans.— B. Sweat glands

211. Ans.— B. Elevated

212. Ans.— E. All of the above

213. Ans.— C. Low leukocyte alkaline phosphatase

214. Ans.— C. Thrombasthenic purpura

215. Ans.— D. High altitude

216. Ans.— A. Myelodysplastic syndrome

217. Ans.— D. Porphyria

218. Ans.— A. Porphyria

219. Ans.— B. ↑ Urobilinogen

220. Ans.— B. G-spike

There is bone marrow failure, amyloidosis, hypercalcemia, pathological fracture etc.

221. Ans.— C. Pigment disappears after treatment with penicillamine

222. Ans.— B. Intracellular crystallization

223. Ans.— C. 280 mosm/kg

224. Ans.— A. CLL

225. Ans.— B. Colonic mucosa

226. Ans.— C. Cu deficiency

227. Ans.— C. Myelophthisic anemia

228. Ans.— A. CML

229. Ans.— C. Beta Chains

230. Ans.— C. Painful and tender

231. Ans.— B. Thalassemia major

232. Ans.— B. Poor release of insulin

233. Ans.— D. ↑ WBC count

234. Ans.— A. Dyshaemopoietic

235. Ans.— C. 69 ml/kg body wt

236. Ans.— D. Bleeding time is increased in idiopathic purpura

237. Ans.— E. 2 : 1

238. Ans.— D. Marfan's syndrome

239. Ans.— C. Chronic constitutional

240. Ans.— A. Infants of drug addicts mothers

241. Ans.— A. This patient has multiple myeloma

242. Ans.— A. Globulin

243. Ans.— C. The urine may be dark and have +ve benzidine test only in the former

244. Ans.— D. None of the above

245. Ans.— B. Centrifugation

246. Ans.— D. Acute myelocytic leukemia

247. Ans.— C. Vit B_{12} deficiency

248. Ans.— A. ITP

249. Ans.— A. Intrathecal methotrexate

250. Ans.— D. Phenobarbitone

251. Ans.— D. All of the above

Serum Iron is raised in —Thalassemia major due to frequent transfusion may lead to Haemosiderosis.

252. Ans.— C. 4 classes are present

253. Ans.— B. Acyclovir-IV

254. Ans.— C. The oxyhaemoglobin dissociation curve is shifted to the left

255. Ans.— B. Decreased neutrophil alkaline phosphatase

256. Ans.— C. ↑ HCL

257. Ans.— B. Vit-B deficiency

258. Ans.— D. Splenectomy

Drugs preferred are interferon or pentostatin or chlorambucil.

259. Ans.— B. Thalassemia

260. Ans.— B. Hypokalemia

261. Ans.— C. The histology is that of nodular sclerosis

262. Ans.— A. 1,2 and 3 are correct

263. Ans.— B. Primary systemic amyloidosis

264. Ans.— B. Hereditary spherocytosis

265. Ans.— C. 2,3 and 4

266. Ans.— B. Sickle cell anemia

267. Ans.— E. Carbamazepine

268. Ans.— C. Corticosteroids

Leukocytosis is caused by corticosteroids and lithium

269. Ans.— A. Steroids

270. Ans.— B. — +

271. Ans.— D.

A	B	C	D
2	3	4	1

272. Ans.— A. Ibuprofen
273. Ans.— B. Salicylates
274. Ans.— B. 30 minutes
275. Ans.— D. Pyridoxine
276. Ans.— C. Azidothymidline therapy
277. Ans.— C. von Willeband's disease
278. Ans.— C. Thalassemia
279. Ans.— B. Spleen
280. Ans.— C. Hemolytic anemia
281. Ans.— A. Liver damage
282. Ans.— C. Mg deficiency
283. Ans.— D. 20%
284. Ans.— C. 70%
285. Ans.— C. - Metabolism of cells
286. Ans.— D. All of the above
287. Ans.— B. Allogenic BM transplant
288. Ans.— A. IgG Kappa Light chain
289. Ans.— D. Anemia
290. Ans.— C. Clot retraction time
291. Ans.— B. Haemosiderin is decreased in bone marrow

Imerslund's syndrome also causes selective cobalamine malabsorption. In blind loop syndrome, bacteria are the cause.

292. Ans.— A. 2 a + 2 b
293. Ans.— D. L-asparaginase
294. Ans.— C. 70-140 microgram

Vit. K is required for clotting factors-II, VII, IX and X.

295. Ans.— A. Soleal vein
296. Ans.— B. Renal failure
297. Ans.— C. ALL
298. Ans.— B. Stuart factor-X
299. Ans.— B. Relative polycythemia
300. Ans.— D. BM transplantation
301. Ans.— D. Urine light chain detection
302. Ans.— B. Clotting time

303. Ans.— B. aPTT

304. Ans.— B. Azotemia

305. Ans.— A. ↓ Serum iron, - serum ferritin, ↓ transferrin

306. Ans.— C. Low molecular weight heparin

307. Ans.— A. Myelofibrosis

308. Ans.— C. Urinary coproporphyrinuria

309. Ans.— C. Decreased platelets in blood

Thrombocytopenia may be caused by drugs such as acetazolamine, aspirin, carbamazepine, carbenecillin, chlorpropamide, chlorthalidone, cotrimexazole, digitoxin, furosemide, gold salts, heparin, indomethacin, INH, Methyldopa, Moxa-lactam, Novobiocin, phenylbutazone, phenytoin (and other hydanloins), quinidine, quinine, thiazides, ticarcillin.

310. Ans.— B. Vitamin-C deficiency

311. Ans.— C. Bolus lignocaine

312. Ans.— A. Lipoprotein (a)

313. Ans.— D. Melphalan

314. Ans.— D. Melphalan

315. Ans.— A. Uroporphyrinogen-III synthetase

316. Ans.— A. Iron deficiency anaemia

317. Ans.— B. Decreased LAP score

318. Ans.— D. Anemia

319. Ans.— C. Aplastic anemia

320. Ans.— B. Serum ferritin

321. Ans.— B. Henoch Schonlein purpura

322. Ans.— B. Candida

Candida is the commonest cause.

323. Ans.— A. Acute leukemia

Blasts are typical of leukemia (especially CML).

324. Ans.— C. Decreased PTT

325. Ans.— C. Increased dose of lignocaine should be given for the procedure

326. Ans.— C. Bence Jones proteins which are excreted in urine are whole immunoglobulin molecule

327. Ans.— A. Multiple myeloma

328. Ans.— C. HbA present reacts allosterically with HbS and prevents HbS from being exposed to low O2 states.

329. Ans.— A. Wegener's granulomatosis

330. Ans.— B. Renal cell carcinoma

331. Ans.— C. Hereditary spherocytosis

332. Ans.— A. Hb 12 g/dL

333. Ans.— A. Iron deficiency

334. Ans.— C. Hypochromic, microcytic anemia

335. Ans.— C. Hodgkin's lymphoma

In early stages of Hodgkin's disease, three areas are used for irradiation—mantle, paraaortic and pelvic.

336. Ans.— C. Thrombocytosis

337. Ans.— C. Antiphospholipid antibody syndrome

Antiphospholipid antibody syndrome may cause renal impairment due to thrombotic microangio-pathy. There are decreased levels of tissue plasminogen activator and increased level of alpha-one antiplasmin.

338. Ans.— B. Bone marrow transplantation

Transplantation from HLA compatible sibling is a curative treatment for aplastic anemia current survival rate is 70-90%. High dose cyclophosphamide with ATG pretransplant immunosuppression and cyclosporine prophylaxis for GVHD (Graft versus Hest Disease) after transplantation has markedly reduced the incidence of graft failure and GVHD.

339. Ans.— A. Sickle cell anemia

Musculoskeletal abnormalities in sickle cell disease are sickle cell dactylitis, joint effusions in sickle cell crises, osteomyelitis, bone infarction, bone marrow infarction avascular necrosis, bone change, secondary to marrow hyperplasia, septic and gouty arthritis.

340. Ans.— A. Thalassemia

341. Ans.— A. Ascites

342. Ans.— B. DDAVP

343. Ans.— B. Chronic myeloid leukaemia

344. Ans.— B. Daunorubicin and cytarabine

345. Ans.— C. Hereditary spherocytosis

346. Ans.— C. Hereditary persistent fetal hemoglobin, homozygous state

347. Ans.— A. Massive lymphocyte apoptosis

348. Ans.— D. Enlarged testis

349. Ans.— A. Tyrosinkinase

350. Ans.— C. 2 and 3

351. Ans.— B. 1 gm%

1 unit = 300 ml.

100 ml blood carry 15 gm Hb.

300 ml blood carry 45 gm Hb

Blood volume for distribution 4.5 litre = 4500 ml

so concentration increase is 1 gm %

352. Ans.— B. Bartonella bacilliformis

Causes of DVT :-

* Bacterial staphylococci, streptococci, meningococci, from negative bacilli.
* Viral : arboviruses varicella, variola, rubella.
* Parasitic-malaria, kala azar,
* Rickettsial : Rocky mountain spotted fever, mycotic: acute histoplasmosis.
* Other causes are clostridia, P falciparum
* Bebsia cause mild haemolytic anemia

353. Ans.— A. Mantle cell lymphoma

* Mantle cell lymphoma is now a well recognized clinical entity that was formerly termed intermediate lymphoma cells are typically of intermediate differentiation.
* The cells express B cell antigens such as CD 19 & CD 20 but also express the nomial T Cell antigen CD5.
* The lack of CD-23 expression.
* Translocation - 11 : 14 brings cyclin D1 under the influence of immunoglobulin heavy chain promoters and leads to cyclin of overexpression.
* Prognosis-Poor

354. Ans.— D. CD_{45} RO

Surface	*Distribution*	*Function*
CD 45 RA	Subset medullary thymocyte (native T cells)	Isoforms of CD 45 Containing Exon 4 (A)
CD 45 RB	All leucolytes Containing Exon 5 (B)	Isoforms of CD 45
CD 45 RC	Subset T medullary thymocyte (native T cells)	Isoforms of CD 45 Containing Exon 6 (C)
CD 45 RO	Subset T cortical thymocyte	Isoforms CD 45 Containing no differentially spliced exon.

356. Ans.— D. Howel-jolly bodies

* **The chronic manifestations of spleenectomy are marked variation in size and shape of erythrocytes (anisocytosis, poikilocytosis) and the presence of Howell-jolly bodies (nuclear remnants)**
* **Heinz bodies - Basophilic stippling and an occasional nucleated erythrocyte in the peripheral blood.**
* **The most serious consequence of spleenectomy is increased susceptibility to bacterial infections, particularly those with capsule, such as Streptococcus penumoniae, Haemophilias influenzae and some Gram negative enteric organism.**

357. Ans.— B. Serum ferritin levels

* **The stored form of Iron in body is serum ferritin so it will be depleted first in Iron deficiency, hence it is the most sensitive & specific marker of Iron deficiency anemia.**
* **Harrison clearly states "The CD2 antigenic molecule is expressed by almost all of the T cells & few non T-cell lineage lymphocytes."**
* **T-lymphocyte function cross links the CD-3/TCR complex or to the T-cell Mitogens which includes Phytohaemoglutinine, Concanavaline A & Pokeweed mitogen.**

358. Ans.— C. Systemic lupus erythematosus.

359. Ans.— C. IgM anti - HBc

360. Ans.— C. Hemochromatosis

361. Ans.— C. Decreased coagulation factor levels

362. Ans.— C. Monoclonal gammopathy of unknown significance

363. Ans.— D. Less than 20,000/mm3

364. Ans.— C. Aplastic anemia

Thrombocytopenia is caused by one of three mechanisms—decreased bone marrow production, increased splenic sequestration, or accelerated destruction of platelets.

Occasional patients have "pseudothrombocyto-penia," a benign condition in which platelets agglutinate or adhere to leukocytes when blood is collected with EDTA as anticoagulant.

The most common causes of immunologic thrombocytopenia are viral or bacterial infections, drugs (often hepatin), and a chronic autoimmune disorder referred to as idiopathic thrombocytopenic purpura (ITP). Patients with immunologic thrombocytopenia do not usually have splenomegaly and have an increased number of bone marrow megakaryocytes.

Cancer chemotherapeutic agents may depress megakaryocyte production. Ingestion of large quantities of alcohol has marrow-depressing effect leading to transient thrombocytopenia. particularly in binge drinkers. Thiazide diurectics.

Most drugs induce thromocytopenia by eliciting an immune response in which the platelet is an innocent bystander.

365. Ans.— D. Clot solubility

The laboratory manifestations include thrombocytopenia and the presence of schistocystes or fragmented red blood cells that arise from cell trapping and damage within fibrin thrombi; prolonged PT and PTT and thrombin time and a reduced fibrinogen level from depletion of coagulation proteins; and elevated fibrin degradation products (FDP) from intense secondary fibrinolysis.

366. Ans.— C. Flow-cytometric analysis

Because the hemoglobin or hematocrit level is affected by the plasma volume, and hematocrit and red cell mass are not linearly related, a red cell mass determination must also be performed to distinguish absolute erythrocytosis from relative erythrocytosis due to a

reduction in plasma volume alone (also known as stress or spurious erythrocytosis or Geisbock's syndrome). Red cell mass determination is important because in polycythemia vera, in contrast to erythropoietin-driven erythrocytosis, the plasma volume is frequently elevated. Masking not only the true extent of red cell mass expansion but often its presence.

Other laboratory studies that may aid in diagnosis include the red cell count, mean corpuscular volume, and red cell distribution width (DW).

Marrow is usually not aspirable due to increased marrow reticulin, but marrow biopsy will reveal a hypercellular marrow with trillineage hyperplasia and, in particular, increased megakaryocytes, but there are no characteristic morphologic abnormalities that distinguish idiopathic myelofibrosin from the other chronic myeloproliferative disorders.

Cytogenetic analysis of blood or marrow is useful both to exclude CML1 and for prognostic purposes, because complex karyotype abnormalities portend a poor prognosis in chronic idiopathic myelofibrosis.

Cytogenetic evaluation in mandatory to determine if the thrombocytosis is due to CML 1 or a myelodysplastic disorder such as the 5q-syndrome. Because the bcr-abl translocation can be present in the absence of the Ph chromosome, fluoroscence in situ hybridization (FISH) analysis for ber-abl expression should be performed in all patients with thrombocytosis rather than a cytogenetic study.

Hematologic Findings : Elevated white blood cell counts, with various degrees of immaturity of the granulocytic series, are present at diagnosis. Usually < 5% circulating blasts and < 10% blasts and promyelocytes are noted. Leukocyte alkaline phosphatase is characteristically low in CML 26 cells.

367. Ans.— B. Add antifungal therapy

Patients with Neutropenia & Fever—Essentials of Diagnosis

* Patients with a polymorphonuclear count of < 500/mm3 or between 500 and 1000/mm3, and is rapidly falling, are at greatest risk of infection.

* Underlying conditions, risk factors, and duration of neutropenia.
* Physical findings that suggest specific microbial etiology of fever with attention to possible foci of infection (e.g. the mouth, lungs, perirectal area, etc).
* Cultures of blood or tissue that yield bacteria, fungus, or virus.

Although up to 90% of patients become febrile during neutropenia, in most cases, fever is the only sign of infection.

Complications :

Superinfection is a recognized complication of febrile neutropenia in patients receiving antimicrobial agents.

A Ub- lactam, either alone or in combination with an aminoglycoside or a fluoroquinolone, is often used.

An acceptable alternative to combination therapy is monotherapy with ceftazidime, cefepime, piperacillin tazobactam, or a carbapenem such as imipenemcilastin or meropenem.

Piperacillin-tazobactam monotherapy is also effective empiric therapy for febrile neutropenia patients.

Ciprofloxacin has a special place in the management of low-risk adult patients as described above.

In patients who remain febrile after 5 days of empiric antimicrobial therapy, antifungal therapy should be added.

The hemotopoietic growth factors G-CSF and GM-CSF are emerging as important adjuvants to the management of neutropenic fever. By increasing the proliferation and differentiation of bone marrow progenitor cells, they help restore neutrophil and macrophage function.

368. Ans.— C. Antibodies to factor-VIII

Thrombotic Disorders

Inherited

Defective inhibition of coagulation factors
Factor V Leiden (resistant to inhibition by activated protein C)
Antithrombin III deficiency
Protein S deficiency
Prothrombin gene mutation (G20210A)
Impaired clot lysis
Dysfibrinogenemia
Plaminogen deficiency
tPA deficiency
PAI-1 excess
Uncertain mechanism
Homocystinuria - endothelial damage
Acquired
Diseases or syndromes
Lupus anticoagulant/anticardiolpin antibody syndrome
Malignancy
Myeloproliferative disorder
Thrombotic thrombocytopenic purpura
Estrogen treatment
Hyperlipidemia
Diabetes mellitus
Hyperviscosity
Nephrotic syndrome
Congestive heart failure
Paroxysmal nocturnal hemoglobinuria
Physiologic states
Obesity
Postoperative state
Immobilization
Old age

369. Ans.— B. Basophils 10-19% of WBC's in peripheral blood
Disease acceleration is defined by the development of increasing degrees of anemia unaccounted for by bleeding or chemotherapy; cytogenetic clonal evolution; blood or marrow blasts between 10 and 20%, blood or marrow basophils = 20%, or platelet count < 100,000/ul. *Blast crisis is* defined as acute leukemia with blood or marrow blasts = 20%. Hyposegmented neutrophils may appear (Pelger-Huet anomaly).

370. Ans.— D. Hairy cell leukemia

This patient has a very typical clinical presentation a 55-year old male, massive splenomegaly and low TLC, which is almost classical of hairy cell leukemia, SLVL usually has a high TLC.

The patient is positive for :

CD19, CD22-Pan B-cell markers

CD-103 Specific for Hairy Cell Leukemia

So, the diagnosis in this case is Hairy Cell leukemia. Other markers positive for Hairy cell leukemia (not in this case) are-CD25, CD11c, FMC-7.

371. Ans.— A Isolated prolonged PTT with a normal PT

Von Willebrand's factor acts as a plasma carrier of factor VIII and circulates in the blood as factor VIII-VWF complex. Its deficiency therefore impairs the intrinsic pathway of coagulation and prolongs the GPTT as the intrinsic pathway of coagulation remains unimpaired, PT is not altered.

372. Ans.— C Henoch Schonlein purpura

'Henoch Schonlein purpura' is the most common of childhood vasculitides with an estimated incidence of 13.5 : 100,000. Pathologically HSP causes a leukocytoclastic vasculitis - Forfur & Arncil's

373. Ans.— C Hb electrophoresis

'The diagnosis of thalassemia syndromes is best established by Hb electrophoresis.'

Thalassemia is a quantitative defect in Hb characterized by lack of certain types of globin chains and compensatory increase in other globin chains. These changes form the basis of electrophoretic investigations and are diagnostic of respective thalassemia syndromes.

Nestroft test : Naked Eye Single Tube Red Cell Osmotic Fragility Test is used for screening of thalassemia but is not diagnostic.

HBAIC : Estimation of glycated haemoglobin is used for estimating long term Glucose control in diabetics. It has no role in thalassemia.

Target cells : May be seen in thalassemia but do not establish diagnosis of thalassemia

Target Cells

Thalassemia

Haemoglobin C, s etc.

Liver diseases

374. Ans. — D. M_3

375. Ans. — D. Hypoploidy

376. Ans. — A. α-thalassemia

377. Ans. — B. Usually are of B-cell origin

378. Ans. — B. Beta thalassemia

379. Ans. — C. Sickle-cell anemia

380. Ans. — D. 0%

* As we know very well that normal HBA2 is 2%
* It increases in case of beta thalassemia major (3.5 to 7.5%)
* It is an AR disorder.
* Genetics - if mother unaffected and father affected so 100% will be carriers but no one will be affected so answer is D.

381. Ans. — D. Aspirin

Low dose aspirin is used prophylactically in cardiac patients or those with stroke to prevent coagulation.

382. Ans. — A. Cephalothin

383. Ans. — C. Erythromboblastosis foetalis

384. Ans. — C. Transfusion reaction

385. Ans. — B. 35 mg bilirubin

386. Ans. — D. Hypokalaemia

387. Ans. — D. Kleihauer test

388. Ans. — D. Chronic myeloid leukaemia

ALL is the commonest malignancy of childhood.

389. Ans. — C. Great sea

390. Ans. — D. Sickle cell anemia

391. Ans. — A. Factor-VIII

392. Ans. — C. 10 gm%

393. Ans. — B. Is the same entity as Henoch-Schonlein purpura

394. Ans. — D. Infant

395. Ans. — C. Henoch-Schonlein purpura

396. Ans. — C. Peripheral smear

397. Ans. — C. Low reticulocyte count

There is reticulocytosis indicating compensatory erythropoisis. Peripheral smear shows polychromasia, burr cells, tear drop cells, spherocytes and fragmented cells.

398. Ans. — B. Idiopathic thrombocytopenic purpura

399. Ans. — C. Oral bleeding

400. Ans. — B. Prevent C N S haemorrhage

401. Ans. — C. Blasts are peroxidase negative

402. Ans. — A. Infection

403. Ans. — C. Vit.-C deficiency

404. Ans. — A. O, Rh negative

O negative is universal donor and AB positive is universal recipient.

405. Ans. — B. 2 months

406. Ans. — D. Ingestion of lead

407. Ans. — D. Iron deficiency

408. Ans. — D. Spread to the meninges unless prophylactic treatment to the central nervous system is given.

409. Ans. — A. Spontaneous haematuria

410. Ans. — C. PTT

411. Ans. — D. WBC around 10000/mm

412. Ans. — C. Breast-fed infants

413. Ans. — A. Autosomal dominant

414. Ans. — D. Phototherapy

415. Ans. — D. ↑ MCH and MCHC

MCH is normal but MCHC is high

416. Ans. — B. Thalassemia

417. Ans. — C. Idiopathic thrombocytic purpura

418. Ans. — D. Splenomegaly

419. Ans. — B. Dapsone

Other drugs implicated are antimalarials, nitrofurans, Sulfas, naphthalene, Probenecid, antipyrin, PAS, nalidixic acid and fava beans etc.

420. Ans. — C. Remits of its own without any treatment in all

421. Ans. — C. Cutaneous porphyria

422. Ans. — C. Lithium

423. Ans. — A. PNH (Paroxysmal Nocturnal hemoglybinuria)
424. Ans. — C. Essential changes involving venous inflammation and subsequent thrombosis
425. Ans. — A. Intrathecal methotrexate
426. Ans. — C. Choice of Treatment-Splenectomy
427. Ans. — A. ITP
In ITP, purpura is not palpable.
428. Ans. — B. B-cell
429. Ans. — B. $\alpha_2\gamma_2$
430. Ans. — A. Mycoplasma
431. Ans. — C. Decreased iron binding capacity
432. Ans. — B. Acute myelocytic leukaemia
433. Ans. — A. Juvenile CML
434. Ans. — D. Anti Lewis
435. Ans. — D. Fanconi's anemia
436. Ans. — B. Methemoglobinemia
437. Ans. — C. Thromboembolism
438. Ans. — B. Sickle cell anemia
439. Ans. — A. 1, 2 and 3 are correct
440. Ans. — B. 7.2
441. Ans. — C. Neuroblastoma
442. Ans. — C. Packed cells
443. Ans. — B. Lead poisoning
444. Ans. — C. Liver
445. Ans. — C. Decreased bone marrow megakaryocytes
Bone marrow shows an increase in number of megakaryocytes which shows diminished budding and have intense blue cytoplasm.
446. Ans. — A. Serum iron estimation
447. Ans. — A. Staphylococcal
448. Ans. — C. HbF
449. Ans. — B. Liver
450. Ans. — C. 70%
451. Ans. — A. Goat's milk
452. Ans. — D. Prolonged bilirubinemia
453. Ans. — A. Sickle cell anaemia
454. Ans. — A. t (8; 22)

455. Ans. — D. Thalassemia and sickle cell trait occuring together

456. Ans. — C. Enteric fever

457. Ans. — D. β_4

458. Ans. — A. Idiopathic

459. Ans. — B. 250—300

460. Ans. — C. More common in formula fed infants

461. Ans. — B. CLL

462. Ans. — A. Leukopenia

463. Ans. — D. Generalised or fulminant gram negative septicemia

464. Ans. — C. Necrotising enterocolitis

465. Ans. — C. Central nervous system involvement

466. Ans. — A. Philadelphia chromosome

Philadelphia chromosome is negative. Chemotherapy is of little help in children.

467. Ans. — D. Vitami-E related anemia

Treatment of choice is venesection and definitive is isovolemic partial exchange with 5% albumin.

468. Ans. — A. Thrombocytopenia

469. Ans. — C. ↑ Adult Hb

There is reduced Erythrocytic count, reticulocytosis, Low MCV, MCH or MCHC, Hypercellular marrow, Erythroblasts in smear, reversed myeloid erythroid ratio and decreased fragility.

470. Ans. — D. ALL

471. Ans. — C. Cord bilirubin —5 mg%

472. Ans. — D. Acute leukaemia

473. Ans. — B. Isoimmune thrombocytopenia

474. Ans. — A. HUS

475. Ans. — A. Hemoglobin electrophoresis

In beta thalassemia, hemoglobin electrophoresis shows only fetal and A2 hemoglobin in children with homozygous beta thalassemia.

476. Ans. — A. SLE

477. Ans. — A. Bone marrow biopsy

478. Ans. — B. 2 months

479. Ans. — D. 200 - 350

480. Ans. — A. Presence of anaemia

481. Ans. — D. Ph (Philadelphia) chromosome

482. Ans. — D. Corticosteroids

483. Ans. — D. All of the above

484. Ans. — A. Serotonin

485. Ans. — D. Normal or increased number of megakaryocytes

486. Ans. — A. Chicken pox

487. Ans. — B. 2—8

Drugs e.g. antiepileptic, cotrimoxazole, PAS, rifampicin, chloromycetin can also produce thrombocytopenia

488. Ans. — A. Usually negative

489. Ans. — D. O -ve cells suspended in AB plasma

490. Ans. — D. Bone marrow examination

491. Ans. — A. Acute leukemia

This child is suffering from acute leukaemia (Presence of splenomegaly exclude the aplastic anaemia and ITP).

Acute Lymphatic Leukemia :

- These are the most common type of childhood malignancy.
- Peak age of onset is 3–7 years.
- More common in male child.
- Bone marrow is replaced by malignant lymphoblast resulting anaemia, thrombocytopenia and granulocytopenia.
- Genetic disease predisposing to leukemia include Down's syndrome, Bloom syndrome, Fanconi's anemia and ataxia telangiectasia.
- The symptoms in order of frequency include fever, petechiae, bleeding, anorexia, malaise and decreased activity.
- Bone pain, arthralgia, hepatosplenomegaly and rarely lymphadenopathy may occur.
- The duration of symptoms may vary from a few days to a few weeks or months at onset
- Bone marrow aspiration or biopsy is needed to ascertain or rule out the diagnosis of acute leukaemia.

Note:

- Liver and spleen are usually not enlarged in aplastic anaemia but are often palpable in leukaemia.
- Spleen is often not palpable in ITP.
- Hypersplenism often not show thrombocytopenia (Petechial spots).

492. Ans. — C. Hemoglobin-D disease

493. Ans. — C. Blood transfusion and desferrioxamine

494. Ans. — A. 14 weeks gestation

An important aspect of human globin genes is regulation of switch from fetal to adult hemoglobin. Beta globin synthesis commences early during fetal life at approximately 8-10 weeks gestation. Subsequently, it continues at a low level approximately 10% of total non-alpha globin chain production, upto 36 weeks gestation after which it is considerably augmented. At the same time gamma globin chain synthesis starts to decline so that at birth there are approximately equal levels of gamma and betta chains produced.

The switch to nearly exclusive synthesis of adult hemoglobin (HbA; $\alpha_2\beta_2$) occurs at about 38 weeks. Fetus and newborn therefore require a globin but not β-globin for normalgestation.

495. Ans. — C. Henoch Schonelin purpura

Henoch Schonelin purpura is the commonest leukocytoclastic vasculitis affecting children.

Leukocytoclastic vasculitis is characterised by a leukocytoclasis, a term that refers to the nuclear debris remaining from the neutrophils that have infiltrated in and around the vessels during the acute states.

Other causes include :

1. Subacute bacterial endocarditis
2. EBV/Infection
3. HIV infection
4. Chronic active hepatits
5. Ulcerative colitis
6. Congenital deficiencies of various complement components
7. Retroperitoneal fibrosis
8. Primary biliary cirrhosis
9. α_1-antitrypsin deficiency
10. Intestinal bypass surgery
11. Relapsing polychondritis
12. Essential mixed cyoglobulinaemia

13. Drug induced vasculitis
14. SLE
15. Rheumatoid arthritis

C/f of leukocytoclastic vasculitis -

Hallmarks of this group of small vessel vasculitis is predominance of skin involvement

The skin lesions appear as -

1. Palpable purpura (Mc)
2. Macules
3. Papules
4. Vesicles
5. Bullae

Other organ system may also be involved

About other options -

1. Polyarteritis Nodosa :
   - Mean age of onset is approx. 50 years of age.
   - It is a necrotizing inflammation of small vessels.
2. Takayascl's disease :
   - Most prevalent in adolescent girls and young women.
   - Inflammatory and stenotic disease of medium and large sized arteries characterized by a strong prediction for aortic arch and its branches.
3. Kawasaki disease :
   - Acute, febrile, multisystem disease of children
   - Immune mediated injury to blood vessel endothelium is the likely pathogenesis involved.

REVIEW PAPER

1. **Macrovalocytosis point towards :**
   A. Alpha thalassemia B. Copper poisoning
   C. Malabsorption D. CLL
2. **Burning of red cells is typically seen in :**
   A. Megaloblastic anemia B. Falciparum malaria
   C. Uremia D. Aplastic anemia
3. **Normal site of haemopoiesis in a 3-months old child is :**
   A. Bone marrow B. Spleen
   C. Liver D. Yolk sac
4. **Active red bone marrow in an adult is maximum in :**
   A. Femur B. Sternum and ribs
   C. Vertebrae D. Pelvic bones
5. **Fat cells begin to appear in the long bones after _____ years of age :**
   A. 2 B. 4
   C. 6 D. 8
6. **One pronormoblast on an average produces ______ erythrocytes :**
   A. 8-10 B. 14-16
   C. 18-20 D. 24-26
7. **Maturation time from pronormoblast to RBC is _____ days :**
   A. 3 B. 5
   C. 7 D. 10
8. **In a pronormoblast, large nucleus occupies ______ % of cytoplasmic space :**
   A. 50 B. 60
   C. 70 D. 80
9. **_________ % of nucleated red cells die in marrow during maturation :**
   A. 2-5 B. 10-15
   C. 20-25 D. 35-40
10. **Normal values for urine erythropoietin in man is _______ units/day :**
    A. 1 B. 2
    C. 3 D. 5

Ans. **1. C** **2. C** **3. C** **4. D** **5. B** **6. B**
7. C **8. D** **9. B** **10. A**

11. **Normal values of plasma erythropoietin have been reported to be _____mU/ml :**

A. 2—5 B. 6—7.5

C. 8.0—9.5 D. 10—12.5

12. **Erythropoietin levels in urine and plásma are increased in :**

A. Fernicious anemia B. Aplastic anemia

C. Leukaemia D. Hypocalcemia

13. **Erythropoietin levels in urine/plasma are _____in polycythemia vera :**

A. Increased

B. Decreased

C. Decreased followed by increased

D. No change

14. **IL-1 is produced by activated macrophages in 2 forms alpha and beta in the ratio of _____:**

A. 1:5 B. 1:10

C. 1:20 D. 1:2

15. **Mature T-cells constitute ______% of circulating lymphocyte population :**

A. 40-50 B. 50-60

C. 65-70 D. 85-90

16. **B-cells comprises ________% of circulating lymphocytes :**

A. 5-15 B. 15-25

C. 25-35 D. 40-50

17. **Median duration of complete circulation is about _______ hours :**

A. 6 B. 10

C. 16 D. 24

18. **PCV is maximum in :**

A. Women B. Full term infants

C. 3 months children D. Children of 10-12 years

19. **Mean cell diameter if erythiocyte is _______μm:**

A. 5.7-5.9 B. 6.1-6.3

C. 6.7-7.7 D. 7.9-9.1

20. **A change in the Hb must be _____g% or more to be considered definitely significant :**

A. 1.0 B. 1.5

C. 2.5 D. 3.0

21. **The ratio of Hb (in gm%) and RBC count per litre is used to calculate :**

A. MCV B. PCV

C. MCH D. MCHC

Ans. **11. B** **12. D** **13. B** **14. B** **15. C** **16. A**
17. B **18. B** **19. C** **20. B** **21. C**

22. **MCV has the normal range of ______ fl :**
A. 50-65 B. 66-76
C. 76-96 D. 96-106

23. **Total body iron is ________ gm :**
A. 2-3.5 B. 3-5
C. 5-6.5 D. 7.5-9.0

24. **Total iron binding capacity is ______ μgm of iron :**
A. 150-250 B. 250-450
C. 400-600 D. 600-750

25. **Red cell proporphyrin is ________ μgm% :**
A. 10-20 B. 20-40
C. 40-60 D. 60-80

26. **Bone marrow iron is ________ :**
A. 1+ to 3+ B. 1- to 3+
C. 1 + to 5+ D. 2+ to 5+

27. **Percentage suburation of transferrin ______ % :**
A. 23 B. 33
C. 40 D. 62

28. **About ______ % of dietary iron is absorbed normally :**
A. 10 B. 20
C. 30 D. 45

29. **Chromium ________ is used to find out life span of RBC's :**
A. 50 B. 51
C. 52 D. 53

30. **Serum iron is normal in ________ anemia :**
A. Iron deficiency B. Chronic infection
C. Thalassemia D. Sideroblastic anemia

31. **Iron in haemoglobin exists as :**
A. Unionised iron atoms B. Ferric irons only
C. Ferrous ions only D. None of the above

32. **The blood concentration of H_2CO_3 (meq/L) is :**
A. 5 B. 15
C. 28 D. 50

33. **The anticoagulant normally present in animal cell is :**
A. Vitamin-K B. Heparin
C. Hyaluronidase D. None of the above

34. **Siderophyllin is :**
A. Haematin B. Ferritin
C. Haemin D. Transferrin

Ans. 22. C 23. B 24. B 25. B 26. A 27. B
28. A 29. B 30. C 31. C 32. C 33. B
34. D

35. **Myoglobin has a molecular weight of :**
A. 12,600 B. 16,800
C. 18,200 D. 24,200

36. **Sulphaemoglobin has a ——— colour :**
A. Cherry red B. Pink
C. Dirty green D. Blue

37. **The colour of choleglobin is :**
A. Red B. Pink
C. Orange D. Green

38. **In comparison to myoglobin, hemoglobin has :**
A. No distal histidine residue
B. More hydrophobic residues units heme pocket
C. Binding sites for more than one ligand
D. A very similar subunit amino acid sequence

39. **Antibodies are which type of globulin :**
A. Alpha B. Alpha-2
C. Beta D. Gamma

40. **Which of the following cells are maximum in normal Arneth count :**
A. One lobed B. Two lobed
C. Three lobed D. Four lobed

41. **Cyclic tetrapyrrole is a synonym of :**
A. Heme B. Porphyrin
C. Hemosiderin D. Bilirubin

42. **Normal volume index of blood is : DNB 1992**
A. 0.4-0.8 B. 0.8-1.1
C. 1.1-1.5 D. 1.5-2.0

43. **Haemoglobin is responsible ———% CO_2 transport in blood :**
A. 40 B. 70
C. 90 D. 99

44. **Ferritin an inactive form of iron is stored in :**
A. Gut B. Spleen
C. Liver D. All of the above

45. **Colour index of blood is :**
A. 0.1-05 B. 0.6-0.9
C. 0.9-1.0 D. 1.0-1.2

46. **Unloading of oxygen to tissue cells by oxy-Hb is assisted by :**
A. Bohr-effect
B. 2-3 diphosphoglycerate
C. Low PO_2 and high PCO_2 in tissues
D. All of the above

Ans. **35. B** **36. C** **37. D** **38. D** **39. D** **40. C**
41. B **42. B** **43. C** **44. C** **45. C** **46. D**

47. **For Haeme synthesis, amino acid required is :**
A. Glycine B. Serine
C. Tyrosine D. Phenylalanine

48. **The anticoagulant, normally present in animal cell is :**
A. Dicoumarol B. Hyaluronidase
C. Vit-K D. Heparin

49. **In normal adult the quantity of haemoglobin catalysed is :**
A. 2 g B. 4 g
C. 8 g D. 16 g

50. **Liver does not produce :**
A. Albumin B. Gamma globulin
C. Fibrinogen D. Prothrombin

51. **Highest binding of iron in plasma is seen with :**
A. Transferrin B. Ferritin
C. Hemoglobin D. Ceruloplasmin

52. **White hair are due to :**
A. Deficiency of melanin
B. High content of iron
C. Increased proportion of Ca and PO4
D. Decreased proportion of calcium carbonate and phosphate

53. **Gamma carboxylation of glutamic acid in clotting factors-II, VII and protein-C is dependent on :**
A. Vitamin-K B. Vitamin-C
C. Vitamin-A D. Vitamin-E

54. **Average amount of total body iron in an adult is ________ gm :**
A. 2 B. 3.5
C. 5 D. 6

55. **When neurological complications are present dose of Vitamin B_{12} in its deficiency states is ______ microgram/d :**
A. 30-100 B. 200-300
C. 300-500 D. 500-1000

56. **Primary indication of erythropoitin in anemia is due to :**
A. Cancer chemotherapy B. AIDS
C. Chronic infections D. CRF

57. **In heparin use, which blood test is used for controlling its dosage :**
A. BT B. CT
C. PT D. All of the above

58. **Which of the following drug may be used as an antidote for heparin :**
A. Vitamin-K B. Hexadimethrine
C. Prothrombin D. None of the above

Ans. **47. A** **48. D** **49. C** **50. B** **51. A** **52. C**
53. A **54. B** **55. D** **56. D** **57. B** **58. B**

59. **Drugs to be avoided in G-6-P-D deficiency are following except :**
A. Dapsone B. Diphenhydramine
C. Phenacetin D. Valproic acid

60. **'Koala Bear' facies may be produced by following foetal teratogen :**
A. Iso-tretinoin B. Ergometrine
C. Phenytoin D. Warfarin

61. **Who gave the name of the 'heparin' :**
A. McLean B. Watson
C. Howett and Holt D. John and Smith

62. **After giving warfarin, the factor whose level falls first is :**
A. VII B. VIII
C. IX D. X

63. **Duration of action of heparin is _____ hours :**
A. 2-4 B. 4-6
C. 6-8 D. 8-10

64. **Epsilon amino-caproic acid (EACA) is an analogue of amino acid :**
A. Methionine B. Leucine
C. Isoleucine D. Lysine

65. **100 ml of blood loss means loss of _______ mg elemental iron :**
A. 15 B. 25
C. 50 D. 75

Ans. **59. D** **60. D** **61. C** **62. A** **63. B** **64. D**
65. C